Research Ethics in Exercise, Health and Sports Sciences

D1258319

Does good research demand good ethics?

Does an emphasis on productivity undermine the moral integrity of research?

Research Ethics in Exercise, Health and Sports Sciences puts ethics at the centre of research in these rapidly expanding fields of knowledge. Placing the issues in historical context, and using informative case studies, the authors examine how moral theory can guide research design, education, and governance. As well as theoretical analysis, key practical concerns are critically discussed, including:

- informed consent;
- anonymity, confidentiality and privacy;
- plagiarism, misappropriation of authorship, research fraud and 'whistleblowing';
- ethics in qualitative research;
- vulnerable populations; and
- trans-cultural research.

Providing an accessible and robust theoretical framework for ethical practice, this book challenges students, researchers and supervisors to adopt a more informed and proactive approach to ethics in exercise, health and sport research.

Mike McNamee is Reader in the Centre for Philosophy, Humanities and Law in Health Care at the University of Wales, Swansea.
Steve Olivier is Professor of Sport and Exercise Science and Head of the School of Social and Health Sciences at the University of Abertay, Dundee.
Paul Wainwright is Professor of Nursing in the Faculty of Health and Social Care Sciences at Kingston University and St George's, University of London.

Ethics and Sport

Series Editors
Mike McNamee, Swansea University
Jim Parry, University of Leeds

The Ethics and Sport series aims to encourage critical reflection on the practice of sport, and to stimulate professional evaluation and development. Each volume explores new work relating to philosophical ethics and the social and cultural study of ethical issues. Each is different in scope, appeal, focus and treatment but a balance is sought between local and international focus, perennial and contemporary issues, level of audience, teaching and research application, and variety of practical concerns.

Also available in this series:

Research Ethics in Exercise, Health and Sports Sciences

Mike McNamee, Steve Olivier and Paul Wainwright

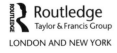

Routledge
Taylor & Francis Group

LONDON AND NEW YORK

First published 2007
by Routledge
2 Park Square, Milton Park, Abingdon, Oxon OX14 4RN

Simultaneously published in the USA and Canada
by Routledge
270 Madison Ave, New York, NY 10016

Routledge is an imprint of the Taylor & Francis Group, an informa business

Typeset in Goudy by
RefineCatch Limited, Bungay, Suffolk
Printed and bound in Great Britain by
TJ International Ltd, Padstow, Cornwall

British Library Cataloguing in Publication Data
A catalogue record for this book is available from the British Library

Library of Congress Cataloging-in-Publication Data
McNamee, M. J. (Mike J.)
Research ethics in exercise, health and sports sciences / Mike McNamee,
Steve Olivier and Paul Wainwright.
     p. cm. – (Ethics and sports)
Includes bibliographical references and index.
1. Physical education and training–Research–Moral and ethical
aspects. 2. Sport sciences–Research–Moral and ethical aspects. 3.
Health education–Research–Moral and ethical aspects. I. Olivier, Steve,
1960– II. Wainwright, Paul. III. McNamee, Mike. IV Title. V. Series.
GV341.M436 2006
174'.961371–dc22
                                                           2006015179

ISBN13: 978–0–415–29881–0 (hbk)
ISBN13: 978–0–415–29882–7 (pbk)
ISBN13: 978–0–203–96685–3 (ebk)
ISBN10: 0–415–29881–4 (hbk)
ISBN10: 0–415–29882–2 (pbk)
ISBN10: 0–203–96685–6 (ebk)

For those who gave us the gift of curiosity, and for those who sustain it

Contents

Series editors' preface

The Ethics and Sport series aims to support and contribute to the development of the study of ethical issues in sport, and indeed to the establishing of Sports Ethics as a legitimate discipline in its own right. It does this by identifying issues of practical concern and exploring them systematically in extended discussion.

Given the logical basis of ethics at the heart of sport as a practical activity, every important and topical issue in sport necessarily has an ethical dimension – and often the ethical dimension is of overwhelming significance. The series addresses a variety of both perennial and contemporary issues in this rapidly expanding field, aiming to engage the community of teachers, researchers and professionals, as well as the general reader.

Philosophical ethics may be seen both as a theoretical academic discipline and as an ordinary everyday activity contributing to conversation, journalism, and practical decision-making. The series aims to bridge that gap. Academic disciplines will be brought to bear on the practical issues of the day, illuminating them and exploring strategies for problem-solving. A philosophical interest in ethical issues may also be complemented and broadened by research within related disciplines, such as sociology and psychology.

The series aims to encourage critical reflection on the practice of sport, and to stimulate professional evaluation and development. Each volume will explore new work relating to philosophical ethics and the social and cultural study of ethical issues. Each will be different in scope, appeal, focus and treatment, but a balance will be sought within the series between local and international focus, perennial and contemporary issues, level of audience, teaching and research application, and variety of practical concern. Each volume is complete in itself, but also complements others in the series.

This volume is a prime example of what the series aims to achieve. The drivers for increased attention to research ethics have been to some extent externally imposed, with the setting up of Research Ethics Committees to monitor proposals for research activity. This has sometimes resulted in a 'box-ticking' approach to the ethical dimensions of research, produced by an inadequate understanding of its nature, rationale and justification, and the generation of an attitude of resigned compliance with what are perceived as irritating yet inescapable bureaucratic requirements.

Part of the work of Ethics Committees in higher education, then, has to be educational – not only in terms of monitoring and improving research proposals, but also in terms of prescribing and monitoring the provision of research ethics education amongst research active staff and amongst undergraduate and postgraduate student populations. As well as serving its function of securing compliance with ethical requirements, it would also be contributing to the development of ethical awareness and understanding amongst its communities of researchers. This volume supplies substantial material for precisely such an education in research ethics.

The authors of this book argue that there is indeed an internal logic at work here that ties ethical competence to research results – that good research exhibits such ethical virtues as will persuade us that we are witnessing genuinely truth-seeking enquiry based on truth-respecting methods, and that the research is deserving of our attention.

For the first time in the context of exercise, health and sports research we find here a systematic and coherent treatment of the salient issues, an application of moral theories and casuistical thinking to commonly occurring cases and contexts, an explication of the possible grounds of decision-making, and an exploration of the role of central concepts, such as anonymity and confidentiality, autonomy, deception, informed consent, plagiarism, responsibility, trust, and more besides. The authors provide a challenge to researchers, teachers and students to reconsider the ethical implications of their research activities, and to us all to re-think our notions of what it is to plan and to execute research in an ethically justifiable manner.

Mike McNamee, Swansea University
Jim Parry, University of Leeds

Preface and acknowledgements

While research ethics in medicine has grown exponentially in the last 30 years it has stuttered along in the fields of exercise, health and sport sciences. In this book, we seek to challenge researchers, students and teachers in these fields, irrespective of their disciplinary research traditions, to take research ethics rather more seriously. Our aim is that it may help to bring about a scenario where research ethics becomes a valued component in research, research methods courses and in the continuing professional development of supervisors and reviewers of research as well.

The authors have been assisted, challenged and supported to provide the text by the help of a multitude of others. It is our pleasure to thank Jacquelyn Allen Collinson, Steve Edwards, Scott Fleming, Malcolm Maclean, Thomas Schramme, Hugh Upton for either reading draft chapters or offering comments and further sources of examples for us.

Samantha Grant and Kate Manson at Routledge have given us excellent service and support along with patient encouragement. Thanks to Andrew Bloodworth for his painstaking formatting of the text and to Keith Thompson for his diligent proof-reading. Finally, a big thanks to Malcolm Willett for his permission to use the cartoon on the front cover.

Introduction

Like all academics today, we three authors carry out a variety of roles: administrator, researcher, supervisor, teacher are among the most common of them. Each of us has also sat on or has been the Chair of University and/ or Local/Multi-Centre Research Ethics Committees for the Public National Health Service. Our ongoing commitment to research ethics has often been in face of *laissez-faire* attitudes (at best) or downright hostility (at worst) to the interference with supposed academic freedoms. Irrespective of the spectrum of researchers' responses to research ethics we have encountered, there is little doubt that in the UK over the last decade or two the pressure to produce and publish research has hit heights previously unknown outside the USA, where 'publish or perish' was the dominant norm for the best part of the twentieth century. Doubtless the drive for accountability with regard to academics' performance is at the heart of the matter and, outside the Academy, this may be thought to be a good thing. What may accompany this drive to performativity and productivity, however, is a variety of attitudes that may undermine the character and conduct of research and researchers.

In this book we try to lay out some of the chief failings of researchers in their pursuit of the truth in exercise, health and sports sciences. We have aimed the text at a variety of audiences: tutors in research ethics and research methods more broadly; active researchers who have failed to consider seriously the ethical dimensions of their research; Institutional Review Board and Research Ethics Committee members whose knowledge of ethics or moral philosophy is lacking or who are unaware of the research traditions beyond their specialism; and of course students at undergraduate and postgraduate levels who are planning their own research.

It is ironic that, in nearly every research methods text in exercise health or sports sciences, even the best of them, there is little more than a few pages (if that) concerned with research ethics. It is as if their authors were so concerned with doing good research – in the technical sense of that word – that the ethical meaning simply escaped their attention. It fell below the radar of research design and designers. Methods matter, morals do not, would seem to be the subtext. Yet, if questioned, these authors, no less than the legion of researchers in these fields, would doubtless proclaim the import-ance of ethics. It might be thought that hypocrisy was the order of the day. Or, in an attempt to be more charitable, one might imagine leaders of the relevant associations saying 'Look, we have codes of conduct' to show that they *really* meant business. As we show in Chapter 1, the most notorious breaches of research ethics of the twentieth century, by the German medical profession, went on while policies governing research conduct were well developed. In this chapter we show, through an admittedly selective and cursory history of research ethics abuses, just why attention to ethical dimensions of research is not to be thought of complacently but rather with a renewed sense of urgency.

While Chapter 1 catalogues a variety of abuses that people can readily recognise as research wrongs, it is another matter altogether to specify pre-cisely why we think of them as wrongful. Many researchers and Institutional Review Board (IRB) or Research Ethics Committee (REC) members will have an intuitive grasp of what is acceptable or unacceptable, permissible or impermissible, virtuous or vicious. Bringing clarity, consistency and coher-ence to these intuitions is a notoriously difficult affair. But it is a crucially important one: for one person's intuition may contrast sharply with another's and, without some kind of rigour to one's moral reflections, the judgements of researchers and their reviewers might seem capricious, subjective or simply relative to any culture, place or time. We reject both relativism and subjectivism.

In Chapter 2 we survey the dominant moral theories of duty-based and consequence-based ethics. We show how moral theory can guide reflection in research ethics. Equally, we show how these considerations are sometimes at odds with each other, even though they share certain formal properties such as their action-guiding, impartial and universalising aims. We also note their inattention to the character of researchers, their moral personality so to speak. We tentatively propose a casuistic approach, which considers, in the absence of strict formulae, moral features of the research as they are salient – whether in terms of benefits, duties, risks and rights – without attempting to reduce the whole of ethical vocabulary to any one criterion such as 'responsibility' or 'integrity'. These noble concepts are certainly not redun-dant, but there is little to be gained by reducing multifaceted problems to singular solutions. Nor will there be any escape from particularising judge-ments according the salience of ethical considerations in the research contexts, as well as paying heed to traditions and precedent. We hope that the chapter will be of particular use to IRB and REC members looking to ground their judgements authoritatively without blind recourse to theory or inflexible method, while avoiding the caprice of subjectivism and relativism.

In Chapter 3 we consider the ethical review of research historically and contextually. We note the critical landmarks in research ethics from the Nuremberg Code to the many versions of the World Medical Association's (WMA) Helsinki Declaration and that of the Committee for International

Organizations of Medical Sciences (CIOMS). We also consider the more local review of research ethics by Institutional Review Boards (predominantly in the USA) and Research Ethics Committees (in the UK). Much of their work is generalisable *mutatis mutandis* with the governance procedures of other countries, and many university-based committees take their lead from these organisations, along with other codes of conduct that are relevant to their disciplinary research traditions. We consider some inherent limitations of all codes of conduct, the aims of which may be as much punitive as educative.

Chapter 4 is the longest and probably the most important chapter of the book. It addresses the complex issue of informed consent – the research ethics notion most widely heard of and probably most widely misunderstood and misapplied. While the first three chapters are more descriptive in nature, this chapter is characterised by philosophical analysis of the various criteria that comprise informed consent. We also consider some frequent – and sometimes unwitting – failures to comply with it. We set out in some detail the moral concept of 'respect for autonomy' on which informed consent is predicated and the paternalistic attitude that it is set against. We outline ways in which certain preconditions as to the voluntariness of the research participant and their comprehension of the research must be met. We also provide considerable detail of what the consent and informational components of informed consent, considered as a process, demand. In so doing we argue against paying lip-service to informed consent, where it is merely viewed as gaining a tick in a box by the researched. We also consider notions such as payment, incomplete risk disclosure and the misuse of gatekeepers to undermine informed consent. Somewhat against our casuistic approach, we conclude the chapter with a checklist of very general considerations that researchers should reflect upon prior to engaging with research participants in the informed consent process.

Many people take it for granted that anonymity, confidentiality and privacy are to be promised at the stage of gaining informed consent. But what this entails, and why these concepts are important though not always necessary, is seldom considered. This is the remit of Chapter 5. All too blithely, researchers often promise that data garnered during the collection process will be treated confidentially and anonymously. Yet, not infrequently, in student research projects, one finds acknowledgements to persons and places which immediately undermine the promises made. Equally, in social scientific or psychological research there is a considerable difficulty in making sense of the context for the reader and not compromising the anonymity of sources. Moreover, in some cases it is all but impossible to hide the identity of the researched and so no promises of confidentiality or anonymity should be made while gaining informed consent. The chapter also considers issues of data collection and storage that make good these promises.

While the varieties of research misconduct are many and various, Chapter 6 goes on to discuss in detail issues of plagiarism and the misappropriation of authorship, which are the most commonly encountered forms of research fraud. We note that cut-and-paste plagiarism – the easiest to perform and punish, is not the only variety, although it may be the one most favoured by students. We note varieties such as the plagiarism of secondary sources and the plagiarism of ideas among others. Their prevalence among researchers is widely suspected though most difficult to prove – a point that goes a long way to proving the necessity of the education of researchers into research that is ethically conceived and practised by strong role models such as mentors or supervisors. Equally widespread, it might be claimed, are abuses of scholarship where authors who are listed play little or no direct part in the production of the research, or whose papers might be written by research sponsors such as pharmaceutical companies. We note relevant advice from journal editors to guide better practice in this area and strongly challenge a widely held assumption that laboratory directors have some kind of right to authorship in virtue of their institutional position. Finally, we consider in this chapter issues of whistleblowing and the potential sanctions against research fraudsters pointing out that their vice is one of injustice: attempting to gain benefits that they are not properly entitled to.

That we have written an entire chapter on ethical issues in qualitative research merits some justification. In our attempt to survey the spectrum of disciplines that comprise research in exercise, health and sports sciences, it will become clear to the reader that critical discussion by scholars is much more deeply concentrated in the areas of health and medicine. This bias has benefits and burdens. On the one hand, many researchers in exercise and sports sciences have always shared strong methodological and ideological interests with biomedical scientists. Why should they not benefit from the fascinating and rigorous debates in clinical and medical research ethics? Of course, our earlier recognition of the importance of contextualising research ethics should warn readers against the simple deduction of norms of research misconduct being applied without reference to social or humanistic sciences.[1] Some of the features of data collection, analysis and reporting are so different in form – in contrast to the rather naïve claims of those who wish to promote some universal 'scientific method' (e.g. Drowatzky, 1996) – that they require particular and practical discussion on their own terms. The myth of the scientific method (Bogen, 2001; Toulmin, 2001) has done much harm in relegating social science to some lower tier ('soft science'), and this denigration may easily seep into an unjustifiably pejorative conception of social scientific research ethics. Nowhere is this more the case than with respect to covert and/ or deceptive research. We discuss the continuum between overt and covert research and also consider – in contrast to the dominant norm of biomedical research – the circumstances in which research *without the informed consent* of the researched may be deemed justifiable and even desirable when other practices such as debriefing and *post hoc* consent are put in place.

In Chapter 8 we deal with the idea of vulnerable populations in research, showing how our treatment of them as researchers calls fundamentally on the virtue of trust. Having set out various categories according to the World Health Organization (WHO), we go on to consider the case of children as the paradigmatic vulnerable population. In this chapter we point out some important inconsistencies between WHO and other international bodies such as CIOMS and national ones such as the Royal College of Paediatrics of Child Health. We also point to some specific difficulties for laboratory-based exercise, health and sports scientists concerning the use of venepuncture in non-therapeutic research where some research appears, despite institutional approval, to have gone against the grain of international research governance in their fields. Stronger still, the very idea of vulnerable populations has come under assault lately and we offer justification for not rejecting but retaining the category, despite the conceptual inflation that has occurred within the lists of those portrayed as vulnerable.

Increasingly, research studies are crossing national and cultural barriers. We discuss the implications of this fact for research ethicists and those wishing to develop their research in accord with respectful practices. One obvious site of contestation is between the individualism of the West and more communitarian culture and politics of other regions of the world. One very practical consequence of this is found in the gaining of consent where it may be extremely disrespectful not to use appropriate gatekeepers or chiefs or community leaders, while relying on the notion of individual autonomy so prized in the West. Equally, simply accepting the dominant norm of the host population should not be taken to imply the consent of those engaged, especially where duress or coercion may be involved. We explore this complex problem, along with others concerning imperialism and distrust, and a hypothetical case study in transcultural research in Chapter 9.

Is bad ethics in research just bad research? Might one say, with impunity, that the science was great but the ethical aspects were ignored or overridden? We argue that research ethics must come to be seen as an essential ingredient in the cake, not merely the icing on the top. We also argue that all research must aim for the benefits that the generation of knowledge can properly bring without ignoring the notion that student research is typically entered into principally for the education of the researcher. Equally, we argue that participation may have its risks but these ought to be reasonable and subject to the consent of the researched.

We hope that each of the populations highlighted above (the ethics board or committee member; the researcher, the research administrator, the student, the supervisor, the teacher of research ethics) will find something of value in these pages. There is always a danger in writing a text for everyone that one will write it for no one in particular. Each of these chapters is relatively free standing. We have not sought to write a book that was, necessarily, to be read from cover to cover. Naturally, our hope is that it will be by all who open its pages, but we are realistic enough to know that the readers will have their own particular interests and their own time constraints. Thus we have allowed a small amount of overlap between chapters so that readers need not constantly refer to other parts of the book.

Our ultimate aim, in the long term at least, is that the book becomes obsolete – not by virtue of being useless, but rather by virtue of its adoption by the various research communities in exercise, health and sports sciences highlighted, and/or by the systematic and substantial inclusion of research ethics in every research methods text hereafter. At least for the time being, then, we hope the text becomes a useful tool for good research and good research education.

1 Why does research need to be regulated?

A selective history of research ethics abuses

The varieties of research, their risks and abuses

It is thought by some that any *normal* adult human being is able to tell right from wrong. What, therefore, could lectures or texts on research ethics really contribute to the conduct of researchers in exercise, health and sports sciences or studies? Surely, it is said, this will be no more than a matter of applying common sense. In the same vein, the sceptic might say that proper conduct in research is a matter of good upbringing and that is the end of the matter. Moreover, those who are possessed of neither good character nor common sense will not be susceptible to lessons in ethics in any case. Such are the hard-nosed views commonly encountered by those committed to research ethics, whether in the roles of colleague, research ethics lecturer or member of Research Ethics Committees.

A number of responses are open to the research ethicist who wishes to combat these sceptical attitudes. They might point to certain codes of conduct which have been developed recently, which attempt to curb the excesses of research misconduct and make clear to would-be researchers that there are penalties that attach to wrongdoing in research. Equally, they might point to the fact that ignorance more than evil is typically the source of harm in research. If this were true, they could argue, then educating people as to those issues that could be avoided by proper planning would constitute worthwhile progress, perhaps even an essential component of students' initiation into research. We prefer to adopt the following strategy: by simply laying before the reader a brief and selective history of abuses in research, the reader will take to be self-evident the case for a compulsory education in research ethics for all researchers in the fields of exercise, health and sports, regardless of whether their disciplinary home is in the natural sciences, the social sciences or the humanities.

The nature and varieties of research and their impact on the scope of research ethics

Before turning to some historical examples of research abuses, it is worth examining the nature of research, and particularly research in exercise, health and sports sciences. As in other areas of scientific inquiry, there has been an ever-increasing demand for research to be undertaken in the sub-disciplines of these areas, from applied anatomy to sports biomechanics and the psychology or sociology of illness and injury. Across these contexts, scientific research is often thought of as critical and exhaustive investigation that has the following aims: (1) the discovery of new facts about the human through systematic observation or experimentation, and (2) the correct interpretation of these facts and the testing of new hypotheses (Christakis, 1992). But this picture is a somewhat skewed one. It is driven typically by what is commonly labelled a positivistic paradigm (see McNamee, 2005: 1–25) and is most clearly exemplified in laboratory research where scientists investigate phenomena in controlled ways in order to find out cause–effect explanations for the occurrence of phenomena.

Though it has yielded vast and important knowledge of the human body and its mental life, it is crucial to bear in mind that this approach to scientific research has been hotly contested on a number of levels. First, it has been challenged by philosophers for claiming a value-free and restrictive definition of science that is neither value-free nor in keeping with developments in the post-positivistic phase of philosophy of science (McNamee, 2005; Parry, 2005). Second, it has been widely argued, by sociologists and psychologists among others, that this definition applies more to quantitative work than to qualitative research, where generalisability is either considered to be less of an issue, or not an issue at all. Gomm (2004: 317), for example, has argued that 'participatory research is usually research which is designed to bring a direct benefit to a small group, and only secondarily to generate knowledge for use by others'. Equally, ethnographers have claimed that the traditional criteria do not apply to unique case studies of local cultures. At the extreme, researchers in autoethnography (Sparkes, 1998, 2000; Allen-Collinson, 2005) claim that central research concepts such as 'reliability' and 'validity' can be used to silence legitimate forms of research that do not conform to the dominant research philosophies and methods. In both of these latter criticisms what is often at stake is the relationship between the scientist and the subject of or participant in,[1] the research. And this brings with it new and interesting ethical issues.

One of these issues, which we consider important to raise at the beginning of this book, lies in the relationship between research and its funding. While it will always be the case, right across the spectrum of scientific study in exercise, health and sports, that some topics are 'hot' or 'sexy' (or just plain old-fashioned), there might well be something more substantive about certain preferences by research funding bodies in relation to types of research. And this might apply as much to internal 'pump-priming' money distributed within a university as it might to large national research funding bodies such as the Economic and Social Research Council (ESRC) in the UK or the National Institutes of Health (NIH) in the USA. If research is not amenable to extrapolation or broader application, or if it cannot be built upon because of unique particularities (i.e. a lot of qualitative research), then support for it is potentially wasteful of public funds. This point is worth noting in order to bear in mind the scope of research and research ethics, which are often thought to be no more than an assembling of technical reminders on how long to keep data, how to avoid exposing identities after having promised anonymity, or which aspects of data protection law to keep an eye on when collecting and reporting findings. Having said this, it is timely to consider the varieties of that thing called research, which will have a bearing on the subject of this book, research ethics.

In considering the nature of research ethics it is necessary, therefore, to begin with a more catholic conception of what research is about. We will take research here to cover all of the following:

- *Basic research*: experimental and theoretical work undertaken to acquire new knowledge of the underlying foundation of phenomena and observable facts, without any particular application or use in view;
- *Strategic research*: applied research in a subject area which has not yet advanced to the stage where eventual applications can be clearly specified;
- *Applied research*: work undertaken in order to acquire new knowledge. It is, however, directed primarily towards practical aims or objectives;
- *Scholarship*: work which is intended to expand the boundaries of knowledge within and across disciplines by in-depth analysis, synthesis and interpretation of ideas and information, and by making use of rigorous and documented methodology;
- *Consultancy*: the deployment of existing knowledge for the resolution of specific problems presented by a client, usually in an industrial or commercial context;
- *Professional practice*: a variant of consultancy applied to certain well-defined professions.[2]

Accordingly, we will refer more generally to these researchers as scientific. We are conscious that this is a diversion from everyday usage of the word 'scientific' but is nonetheless very much in keeping with European usage of the word, where it is used to denote the development of knowledge according to well-understood techniques and traditions but not merely those that are experimentally focused. Under this loose conception, philosophy is a science and so is sociology. They merely represent disciplined and rigorous ways of coming to know about ourselves and the world. Where a specific research tradition is being focused upon we will adopt the practice of including a qualifier such as 'experimental', or 'natural scientific', or 'case study' as a predicate.

One important caveat should be noted here because it has significant implications for the ethical demands placed upon it: this is the distinction between therapeutic and non-therapeutic research. Research is said to be therapeutic if it is potentially of direct benefit to the participant(s), and non-therapeutic if it is not intended to be of direct benefit to the patient or normal volunteer. So in non-therapeutic research the participant does not necessarily benefit, and may be inconvenienced or even harmed. Most health and, indeed, much sports medicine research falls into this category.[3] Whatever the terminology, we need to be aware that research is not necessarily therapeutic and that assumptions to the contrary carry risks for researchers and participants. There is perhaps a human tendency to overrate the benefits and underestimate the risks of research, particularly where therapy is involved, and researchers need to guard against even unwittingly exposing research participants to unreasonable risks (Capron, 1989). The nub of the problem is captured particularly well by Katz:

> When may a society, actively or by acquiescence, expose some of its members to harm in order to seek benefits for them, for others, or for society as a whole?
>
> (Katz, 1993: 34)

This precise question needs to be asked not only in the contexts of the role of scientific research and scholarship, but also in the light of prevailing and conflictual ethical theories. We shall leave the latter task until Chapter 2 but will consider the former immediately.

Research, ethics and society

Free scientific inquiry and social stability have often been at odds, and the interface between scientists and the public has historically been beset with conflict. For confirmation, one has only to turn to the example of Galileo. Many social and political concerns have consistently produced, and continue to produce, friction between scientific inquiry and societal concerns. The issue of genetically modified athletes, for example, produces heated debate, as does the issue of cloning and research with any potential impact on medical conditions and on sports performance. Particularly when research (and the freedom to conduct it) impinges on the perceived rights of individuals or groups, a sense of alarm grows even in societies that have traditionally given free rein to such activities (Bok, 1978a: 19).

In exercise, health and sports sciences, progress has demanded that subjects be increasingly subjected to manipulative, and sometimes even invasive, methods or techniques. For example, invasive procedures may involve the researcher taking blood samples and biopsies, using radioactive tracers, requiring the subject to exercise to maximum effort, penetrating deep into a given subculture or performing potentially invasive psychological interventions. The diverse nature of research means that while procedures may be carefully implemented and controlled, the specific effects cannot be predetermined with unhesitating confidence. Control is very much a metaphor for experimental research and has been since Sir Francis Bacon's seventeenth-century foray into the empirical sciences. Nevertheless, while accepting tensions inherent in situations involving new research techniques, in Western society, science plays a revered role, and scientific development has long been regarded as a relatively undisputed good for everyone. For example, Western medicine, a fundamentally rational and experimental branch of applied science (at least in its dominant modern conception), holds research in high esteem and bases much of its power on it. Macilwain (1996) argues that the American public at least continues to hold science in respect, with three-quarters of the population believing that the benefits of research outweigh its harmful results. As noted above, it is more than unlikely that the questionnaire respondents from whom the data were collected had any kind of critical appreciation of the complex and contested nature of scientific inquiry. We can concede, however, that research in these contexts is not without risks and, particularly as a result of problems arising in the medical arena, ethical issues have recently exploded into the public consciousness.

The current awareness of ethical issues has led to some doubt as to whether research, particularly research involving human subjects/participants, is based on shared interest, between researcher and object, between society and researcher, and between society and the individual, or whether certain areas of research contain different or even antagonistic interests (Scocozza, 1989).

This raises the issue of whether or not current research practices are geared towards particular theories of ethics. There is no dominant theory of ethics that is agreed upon by philosophers, let alone by natural or social scientists. Three dominant theories will be dealt with in Chapter 2. Briefly, however, we can denote their shape here as a first sketch. First, virtue theory encourages persons to behave in ways that we would recognise as 'good' (e.g. courage, fairness, honesty, impartiality). Virtue theorists do not seek to directly answer the question 'What should I do here?' but instead focus on the kinds of person (here: researcher) that it is desirable to be. Doing the right thing will necessarily flow from being the right kind of person. Second, utilitarian ethics are characterised by the importance they attach to the overall benefits or utility of the acts that one performs. In a research context this means that ethical acceptability is assessed on the basis of the consequences, specifically the applicability of the results (Scocozza, 1989). In short, utilitarians contend that the ethically defensible is that which can be beneficial to the greatest number of people. Third, deontologists (or duty-based ethicists) maintain that ends do not justify means and that an individual's interests, freedom and possibility of choice must be central. The respect that we owe others, especially research subjects and participants, is understood as a catalogue of duties that we have towards them.

Which approach holds sway in our current research environments? Brodie and Stopani (1990) have little doubt that the utilitarian view tends to predominate in experiments in natural scientific research in exercise and sports, and this supports the view held by Rifkin (1988), Scocozza (1989) and Evans and Evans (1995), who similarly contend that the predominant ethics within the health sector are utilitarian. The quest for knowledge about the human body and mind has further resulted in researched populations being increasingly subjected to invasive, intrusive, potentially dangerous experimentation, and this has, in some cases, led to harmful consequences. As we shall see, the history of research provides abundant evidence to show how easy it is to exploit individuals. This is particularly the case when the only moral guide for science is a naive utilitarian dedication as to the greatest good for the greatest number (Fethe, 1993).

Utilitarian ethics are thought to be a natural or sometimes inevitable result of a positivist approach to science. This approach is criticised by French (1987: 18), who states 'In the positivist programme, research is something that is done to people, perhaps for people, but the stance of objectivity prevents it from being done together with people or by them.' Implicit in this approach then, as we noted above, is an epistemological approach with ethical implications. Note that participatory research, such as action research or certain approaches to feminist research, is designed to be for and with the participants (as opposed to subjects) and not merely on them. This is why the terms 'subject' and 'participant' are not inert but powerfully loaded terms that clarify the presuppositions of the researchers themselves.[4] Indeed, there is an ethical imperative in doing sound research, for otherwise social change will be left in the hands of people who are unable to substantiate their ideas on the basis of reliable evidence (Blanck et al., 1992). Nevertheless, as Bok observes, 'If total harmlessness were a prerequisite, little progress would be made in areas where urgent needs must be met' (1978: 124).

Research ethics as risk regulations

One persisting voice of the scientific lobby, perhaps more specifically in natural sciences, is the idea that science somehow exists in a moral vacuum. It is thought by some that, rather like the law, it is neither moral nor immoral but amoral. So scientists should be allowed to pursue their research agenda unfettered by moral considerations as long as they follow the accepted norms of valid scientific research. Sometimes to this position is added the rider that the generation of new knowledge concerning ourselves and the world is of supreme intrinsic value and should trump other concerns. Yet historically there have been, and continue to be, numerous demands for the regulation of research with injurious or invasive potential. As Bok summarises: 'The freedom of scientists to pursue research unchecked must ... be weighed against the freedom of those affected by the research' (Bok, 1978a: 15). Following on from this, the risk of retarding progress and hampering researchers through regulation must, in turn, be weighed against the risk of harm in the absence of regulation.

Many in what is all too loosely called the scientific community would probably be disturbed that the question even arises. They probably contend that, generally speaking, the risks are relatively small or non-existent and, further, when there are significant risks, the researcher's integrity and the existing avenues of regulation are sufficient to provide adequate protection for research participants.

Some of these claims are of course legitimate. Many researchers in exercise, health and sports domains pursue tasks so benign that they are not even remotely capable of threatening anything or anyone. It is not always the case that the apparently unproblematic can have consequences of significant ethical import. One example might be questionnaire administration to examine attitudes to daily exercise and nutrition in schools. In cases such as this, it might be thought – particularly if coercion is absent and anonymity guaranteed – that consent is implied by mere participation as refusal to reply is a viable option. What might happen, however, if a damning set of responses were recorded as to the perceived nutritional content of school dinners? What might happen in a round of redundancies if it became clear that a given teacher deliberately interpreted curricular requirements towards elite sports coaching rather than including health-related exercise as prescribed? This is not to say that much research is morally mundane. It is simply to highlight how apparently innocuous research can have very serious consequences when data thought to be for one purpose is used for another, and in a way that neither researcher nor the researched could have foreseen.

It is difficult however to classify certain *types* of research as potentially harmful and others as risk-free. For example, even observational studies, in themselves seemingly least capable of having an effect of a harmful nature, can carry risks through improper and intrusive observation. Also, when observation takes the place of known therapy, as in the Tuskegee study (see p. 21), the very lack of action is considered unethical. There is no neat dividing line, and were such a barrier to be suggested it would have to be considered an artificial one.

Nevertheless, the point is that many researchers, if they consider the issue at all, view their investigations as fundamentally risk-free. Of greater significance though is that others, who do perceive some threats from certain kinds of research, may consider the potential benefits to humanity as sufficient compensation, which is of course a consequence-driven (utilitarian) approach. It may of course be legitimate to argue that certain risks are unavoidable and necessary if society is to gain from research, but here it becomes important to raise issues of distributive justice. For example, Bok (1978a: 117) states that: 'It is no accident that much research of a questionable nature has been conducted on the most vulnerable and helpless: on children, the institutionalised, the sick and the poor.'

On determining risk and benefit in research

If it is true that particular attention needs to be paid to contexts where risks can be foreseen or with regard to populations who are in and of themselves, at risk, what, precisely, do we mean by these terms? The term 'subject at risk' has been defined to mean:

> Any individual who may be exposed to the possibility of injury, including physical, psychological, or social injury, as a consequence of participation as a subject in any research, development, or related activity which departs from the application of those established and accepted methods necessary to meet his needs, or which increases the ordinary risks of daily life, including the recognized risks inherent in a chosen occupation or field of service.
>
> (Department of Health, Employment and Welfare [DHEW], 1978, in Liemohn, 1979: 158)

Further, if an investigation is for the sole purpose of benefiting the subject, the subject should be considered at risk if any biological, emotional or behavioural condition is investigated (Liemohn, 1979). More recently, the Code of Federal Regulations holds that risks should be minimised[5] through sound research design, avoidance of exposure to unnecessary risks and, where possible, the use of procedures already performed on the subjects for diagnostic or treatment purposes. Of course, different types of research will pose different types and possibilities of risk, and many experiments may not involve risk beyond that experienced in ordinary life situations (see note 5). However, this does not relieve the investigator of the responsibility for protecting research participants. Most codes include early on the idea that, irrespective of the existence of professional regulations, it is ultimately the responsibility of the researcher to ensure that the research is conducted in an ethically acceptable manner.

In much research there is in fact little clear abuse, though the magnitude and probability of potential risks is very often disputed. Equally, however, the benefits hoped for are often conjectural. A widely accepted idea in health and medical research is that the research should aim toward demonstrable benefits which attach to a population beyond the researcher where the $n = 1$. Applying this norm, then, one must be sensitive to the level at which the research is being carried out. Very often undergraduate research will not satisfy this condition strictly, yet with no reasonable prospect of harm one would not expect the researcher to be denied the ability to carry it out. To use the title that derives from this principle: research should be beneficent. Nevertheless, Research Ethics Committees are typically exhorted to (a) ascertain if research increases risk beyond an acceptable level and (b) determine the 'risk–benefit' ratio.

As a general norm, it is safe to say that in research contexts the idea of 'benefit' should be conceived of as the benefit to science from an increase in generalisable knowledge, as well as for specific populations with whom the research is conducted. This again introduces the question of utility, and the willingness of society to accept such benefits – even perhaps at the expense of unwilling individuals – needs to be borne in mind when evaluating the legal and ethical issues posed by research (Capron, 1989).

The above arguments are largely conjectural. The sceptic is likely to say that this is a storm in a teacup. 'Are there in fact any *real* risks associated with research in exercise, health and sports?', they might reasonably ask. In a retrospective analysis of empirical studies of injuries to research subjects, Cardon *et al.* (1976) found injuries were reported for 0.7 per cent of 133,000 subjects; 80 per cent of these injuries were classified by the principal investigator as trivial, and nearly all the remainder as temporarily disabling. Permanently disabling and fatal injuries together accounted for about 1 per cent of all injuries. When distinguishing between therapeutic and non-therapeutic research, of 93,000 subjects who participated in non-therapeutic studies, 0.8 per cent were reported injured, indicating in general that non-therapeutic research is much safer than some types of therapeutic research.

It is also worth recognising that a large majority of immediately identified injuries that occur in therapeutic research are well-recognised hazards of the treatment/s employed. In evaluating the results, Cardon *et al.* (1976) conclude that the risks of participation in non-therapeutic research may be no greater than those of everyday life, and in therapeutic research, no greater than those of treatment in other settings.

Virtually any study produces some risk, and consequently it is the task of the investigator (and the Ethical Review Board) to establish whether or not the risks present are significant ones. Would the taking of a blood sample, which always carries the risk of a haematoma, be considered a significant risk? Many exercise laboratories do cholesterol screening, or assess haemoglobin levels, using simple finger-prick devices. Kroll (1993) reports that these have a known risk of hepatitis B transmission, to the extent that in the USA the Food and Drug Administration (FDA) released a nationwide alert about improper use of such devices.

Can we really determine the potential risks of exercise tests? Kroll (1993) reported the American College of Sports Medicine (ACSM) position that, having weighed the risk of death against the benefits of exercise, the overall risk–benefit ratio for an active way of life is favourable. This is justified by the fact that, while death rates are transiently increased during the test, they are presumably decreased for the remainder of the day. Specifically, a slightly higher risk of cardiac arrest of 21 events per 100 million person-hours during exercise compared to 18 events in sedentary men is considered reasonable. Nevertheless, the ACSM informed consent example for a health-related exercise test also includes a statement regarding the following risks: abnormal blood pressure, fainting, disorder of heartbeat and, in rare instances, heart attack, stroke or death. Also, to facilitate safe exercise testing and prescription, the organisation suggests pre-participation screening for risk factors and contra-indications to exercise (Guidelines for Exercise Testing and Prescription, 2006: 19).

Kroll (1993) reports a study which found a mortality rate of 1 per 10,000 tests, and a combined mortality–morbidity rate of 4 per 170,000 tests. This is contrasted with a death rate of 0.5 per 10,000 exercise tests reported by the ACSM at the time (Kroll, 1993). More recent figures (Guidelines for Exercise Testing and Prescription, 2006) are estimated as 1 death per year for every 133,000 men and 769,000 women, respectively, during or within one hour of exercise participation for high school or college athletes. It is worth noting that regular physical activity reduces the risk of atherosclerotic cardio-vascular disease, but vigorous exertion also transiently increases the risk of sudden cardiac death where there is pre-existing heart disease (Guidelines for Exercise Testing and Prescription, 2006). So, regardless of precautions taken, it is difficult to completely eliminate the risk of a serious event during exercise testing or participation.

Turning briefly to the issue of risk–benefit ratio, Kroll (1993) states that intrinsic to informed consent, particularly in a medical context, is the assumption that the clinical treatment of a research subject would surpass the benefits associated with a traditional treatment regimen. Additional possible risks have also to be factored into the equation, however, and if the new treatment had significant risks with only slightly increased benefits, the proposed investigation might be deemed inadvisable. This has some relevance in the use of control groups in exercise regimen investigations, which typically involve comparison of new techniques against traditional ones, i.e. the control group.

While the control group would not be subjected to any additional risks, are there in fact any benefits attached to their participation? In tests where the control group is subjected to a traditional exercise regimen, for example, they clearly do derive some benefit. However, when a control group is required to remain sedentary, are they being treated ethically? Though it may be true that they accrue no additional risks, we ought still to ask whether they are receiving any benefits from participation in the study. If, following assessment, subjects are considered 'at risk' according to US Code of Federal Regulations, the following conditions must be met for a research project to receive approval:

(1) Risks to subjects are minimized: (i) By using procedures which are consistent with sound research design and which do not unnecessarily expose subjects to risk, and (ii) whenever appropriate, by using procedures already being performed on the subjects for diagnostic or treatment purposes.

(2) Risks to subjects are reasonable in relation to anticipated benefits, if any, to subjects, and the importance of the knowledge that may reasonably be expected to result. In evaluating risks and benefits, the IRB should consider only those risks and benefits that may result from the research (as distinguished from risks and benefits of therapies subjects would receive even if not participating in the research). The IRB should not consider possible long-range effects of applying knowledge gained in the research (for example, the possible effects of the research on public policy) as among those research risks that fall within the purview of its responsibility.

(3) Selection of subjects is equitable. In making this assessment the IRB should take into account the purposes of the research and the setting in which the research will be conducted and should be particularly cognizant of the special problems of research involving vulnerable populations, such as children, prisoners, pregnant women, mentally disabled persons, or economically or educationally disadvantaged persons.

(4) Informed consent will be sought from each prospective subject or the subject's legally authorized representative, in accordance with, and to the extent required by §46.116.

(5) Informed consent will be appropriately documented, in accordance with, and to the extent required by §46.117.

(6) When appropriate, the research plan makes adequate provision for monitoring the data collected to ensure the safety of subjects.

(7) When appropriate, there are adequate provisions to protect the privacy of subjects and to maintain the confidentiality of data.

  (b) When some or all of the subjects are likely to be vulnerable to coercion or undue influence, such as children, prisoners, pregnant women, mentally disabled persons, or economically or educationally disadvantaged persons, additional safeguards have been included in the study to protect the rights and welfare of these subjects. Why does research need to be regulated?

Detailed guidelines regarding risk–benefit assessment, and classification of risks (e.g. negligible, minimal, more than minimal), exist, but it could be argued that, whatever the perceived benefits to mankind in general, harmful or careless treatment of subjects is never justified. This is consistent with Zelaznik's (1993) contention that the use of human subjects in research is a privilege, and the rights of research participants always outweigh the desires of the researcher to conduct research.

Ethical issues in qualitative work are dealt with comprehensively in Chapter 10, but it is worth mentioning here that qualitative projects are not without risks simply by virtue of their nature. Principally, risks in qualitative research surround the possibility of social or psychological harm where confidentiality or anonymity has not been preserved. Material harm is also possible, for example in occupational studies, such as the perception of quality of working environment, where inadvertent disclosure of sensitive information gathered in a study may seriously prejudice career prospects.

Given the very nature of research, it is not always easy to predetermine the presence and extent of risk in any given investigation. Nevertheless, the effort to identify these features of the research responsibly is a critical feature of good research design. Despite the grandiose claims of certain scientists, it is as well to remember that progress is an optional not a mandatory goal, and its pursuit must take place within limits established by other values, including the value of individual autonomy (Capron, 1989). The effort to identify risks in research must be constant (Bok, 1978a), and ethical scrutiny is needed to determine the cost of research, when cost includes possible harm to values other than the advancement of knowledge (Capron, 1989). This introduces the point of view that researchers should consider the moral stance that the rights of the study participant ought always to outweigh the desires of the researcher to conduct research (Zelaznik, 1993; Olivier, 1995).

Risks and regulations

Why is there such a seemingly strong perception of potential risks inherent in research? The current legislative and regulatory research ethics environment has its antecedents primarily in a reactive response to history.

Essentially, the regulation of research became inevitable as a response to abuses perpetrated on humans in the name of research, under the guise of advancing our knowledge. By the turn of the twentieth century, biomedical research was a growth industry. The public demand for knowledge seemed insatiable. Vaccines against diseases, coronary bypass surgery, organ transplantation and so on, all resulted from human or animal experimentation. With experimentation increasing exponentially, scandals were inevitable. What follows are a few selective but well-known examples of controversial projects that contributed to calls for better regulation of research.

The utility of knowledge: at what cost?

We noted above that some scientists claim that the expansion of human knowledge is in itself sufficient to justify scientifically valid research. This is not a position that finds much assent among researchers these days. Rather, as we have suggested above, responsible researchers should make serious efforts to identify reasonably the risks and benefits of their research in some tangible way so that an estimation of costs and benefits can be made. Much has been undertaken in political spheres in the name of human progress and it is no surprise that health-related research has often been involved.

One early case of abuse in this vein occurred in 1916 when Wiles inoculated rabbits with the treponenes that cause syphilis, which he had obtained by trephining (opening) the skulls of six insane patients and by taking a small sample of their brain. As with other experiments, the intention was find a cure to ultimately benefit humankind. Nevertheless, the ethical issues surrounding the work (in this case the use of vulnerable patients) raised questions about the moral climate in which the experiments were conducted. While defending the research, the American Medical Association recognised that there was a need to establish ethical guidelines for research (Pettit, 1992).

Similar experiments were conducted in Germany in the 1920s and, as a result of public and professional outrage, ethical guidelines were formulated. For example, the existing Prussian regulations were superseded by a new set of German rules in 1931 (the *Richtlinien*). The official response to public concern focused, as did later responses, on two issues: that of the risk of harm, and informed consent (BMA, 1992; Pettit, 1992)

Previous and subsequent regulatory mechanisms have, however, emphasised the need to control the risks presented to subjects by research, rather than to enable autonomous choice to participate in research (Faden and Beauchamp, 1986). The issue of freely agreeing to participate in research, in the full knowledge of its nature, purposes and risks, has been taken to be the crucible of most research ethics and is discussed in detail in Chapter 4. Nevertheless, both considerations are central themes in the history of the application of ethical thinking in research contexts.

Despite the examples above, there was little further interest in issues such as informed consent prior to the Second World War. Current concerns with subject autonomy grew gradually after what could be considered a series of watershed events, namely the unprecedented cruelties administered by scientist-physicians during the Nazi regime in Germany. These events were to trigger the changes in how we currently view the involvement of human participants in research (Faden and Beauchamp, 1986).

Before describing some of the experiments conducted by Nazi scientists, it is important to note that the 1931 German *Richtlinien* governing research on humans were stringent and exhaustive. For example, questions of the nature of appropriate information, bona fide consent, careful research design and special protection for vulnerable subjects were all included. Consent was mandatory for human experimentation, and laboratory and animal experimentation had to be completed before human involvement could be considered (Faden and Beauchamp, 1986; Capron, 1989).

So stringent regulations were in place to promote ethical conduct in research. The abuses perpetrated are thus all the more remarkable for their occurrence, and this illustrates that regulations and official endorsement are not sufficient conditions for protecting research participants (Olivier, 1995). Put differently, rules are necessary, but they are not enough to ensure good conduct in research. What else is needed? Perhaps a virtuous character on the part of researchers? Perhaps a consideration of the rights of research participants? Perhaps a calculation that the benefits of a project outweigh the risks? Or perhaps a judicious mix of all of these. In any event, despite the regulations in place, the Nazi experimenters ignored both of the central themes mentioned earlier, namely beneficence and autonomy (Annas and Grodin, 1992).

Research subjects were most often drawn from those incarcerated in concentration camps. Voluntary consent requirements were ignored. Research activity in some cases centred on helping the 'war effort'. For example, some studies simulated low-pressure environments to examine the human response to high altitudes such as would be encountered by pilots. Many subjects died in these experiments.

Further research included experiments where prisoners were deliberately wounded. The subjects' condition was then aggravated by procedures such as the tying off of blood vessels to produce gangrene, by deliberate infection with bacteria such as streptococcus, or by forcing ground glass or wood shavings into the wound to test the effectiveness of different drugs. Sulfanilamide, for example, was then administered to fight the infections, with the reactions being monitored.

In other studies subjects were used as human incubators – prisoners were intentionally infected with jaundice or typhus and then tracked via various research protocols. Gasoline, sea-water, and various poisons were administered to subjects intravenously and orally, and autopsies conducted on those who died. Others were killed intentionally for autopsy purposes, for example sets of identical twins. It is still not clear how many people died, but it is estimated that approximately 1,750 Jewish, Russian, Polish and gypsy prisoners were involved (Faden and Beauchamp, 1986; Capron, 1989; Kroll, 1993).

Perhaps most notorious were the hyperthermia experiments of Dr Sigmund Rascher and colleagues, which were reported by Dr Franz Blaha, a Czech doctor who became an inmate at Dachau in 1939. His transcript at the Nuremberg trials reads:

> The subject was placed in ice-cold water and kept there until he became unconscious. Blood was taken from his neck and tested each time his body temperature dropped one degree. . . . The lowest body temperature reached was 19 degrees centigrade but most men died at 25 or 26. When the men were removed from the icy water attempts were made to revive them with artificial sunshine, hot water electrotherapy, or by animal warmth. For this last experiment prostitutes were used and the body of the unconscious man was placed between two such women.
>
> (Godlovitch, 1997: 2)[6]

Horrific experiments were not confined to Nazi scientists. Between 1930 and 1945, under Japan's biological warfare programme, a group called Unit 731 conducted experiments on Chinese prisoners-of-war in occupied Manchuria. The facility was capable of producing 8 tons of bacteria per month, and experiments on humans included prolonged exposure of the liver to X-rays, freezing body parts to try various methods of thawing, infusing horse blood into the body and vivisection. Also, experiments were conducted on the human response to anthrax, botulism, cholera, dysentery, smallpox, syphilis, typhoid and typhus. It is speculated that at least 3,000 people were killed in these experiments, and that several other similar research units were in existence at the time (Capron, 1989).

Prosecution and conviction as per the Nazis was not the fate of these Japanese researchers. In exchange for not being publicly tried and punished, they agreed to cooperate and share their results with officials of the USA, who adopted a baldly utilitarian standpoint upon discovery of the unit and its activities. This stance in itself is highly problematic (Godlovitch, 1997). They protected the researchers from prosecution and justified this on the grounds that the value of the information far outweighed the value of prosecution. The reasoning was that the findings greatly augmented scientific knowledge and were unobtainable elsewhere because of more stringent controls on human subject research (Capron, 1989).

Recent health-related research transgressions

Harmful experiments were not confined to solving questions arising from war, nor were they confined to a particular group of nations. In the United Kingdom, human testing was carried out at Porton Down in the 1950s as part of British and American attempts to develop chemical weapons at the beginning of the Cold War. The nerve gas Sarin was placed on the skin of human volunteers and one person died, with others suffering adverse reactions. It is claimed that the servicemen 'volunteers' were deceived into thinking that they were taking part in experiments to find a cure for the common cold.

In 1932 the US Public Health Service commenced a study that involved monitoring the condition of untreated syphilis in a population of rural black males near Tuskegee, Alabama. No consent was obtained, the subjects were kept in complete ignorance of the experiment, and they were actively discouraged from seeking or receiving effective treatment, lest that interfere with the data (Capron, 1989). Even after 1945, when penicillin was known to be a safe and effective cure, the Department of Health, Education and Welfare failed to practise its own stated research safeguards and continued the study with an untreated control group. The study was only terminated in 1972 (Kroll, 1993). In 1997, the then President of the USA, Bill Clinton, issued a public apology on behalf of the government for the way in which the study was conducted, at the same time extending the charter of the National Bioethics Advisory Commission.

Public awareness of the need for protection of human subjects was also heightened in 1962 by reports of research at the Jewish Chronic Disease Hospital (JCDH). The chief researcher, Chester Southam, persuaded the JCDH medical director, Emmanuel Mandel, to allow research involving the injection of a suspension of live cancer cells into 22 geriatric patients who

were not suffering from cancer. The motivation for the research was to dis-
cover whether in cancer patients a decline in the body's capacity to reject
cancer transplants was caused by their cancer or debilitation, and it was
hypothesised that each patient would reject the injected cells (as a matter of
biological law) because they are foreign. Thus it was argued that no patient
was at increased risk of developing cancer as a result of the injections.
Although some patients were allegedly given some oral information regarding the experiment, no consent was obtained, and no one was told that they
were being injected with cancer cells. Following the controversy surrounding
the case, in 1966 the Board of Regents of the State University of New York
censured Southam and Mandel, deploring their utilitarian assumptions
regarding research, their disregard for subjects' rights, and the manner in
which deception was practised (Faden and Beauchamp, 1986; Pettit, 1992;
Kroll, 1993).

In 1966 Henry Beecher took an important step towards heightening
awareness of moral problems in research by conducting a literature search of
major medical journals. His findings, reported in the *New England Journal of
Medicine*, highlighted 50 cases of ethically dubious research, with subject
consent being obtained in only two of these cases. The research cited
included the withholding of effective treatment. In one case this resulted in
the deaths of 23 patients from typhoid. Beecher argued that even if only a
quarter of the studies cited were truly unethical, this was still indicative of a
serious situation (see Faden and Beauchamp, 1986).

Beecher also cited the work of Pappworth who revealed numerous
examples of maleficence and deception in research. Many of these experiments were performed on newborn infants, children, pregnant women, surgery patients, the mentally handicapped and the dying. The experiments
generally involved persons whose consent was difficult or impossible to
obtain. Pappworth concluded that researchers often take risks with uninformed subjects in situations where full disclosure of information would
probably result in non-participation (Faden and Beauchamp, 1986).

A further major controversy developed at a New York institution for the
severely retarded, Willowbrook State School. The school was overcrowded,
and unhygienic conditions prevailed. In attempts to develop a vaccine for the
hepatitis virus that a large percentage of the children contracted, Saul Krug-
man and his associates deliberately infected newly admitted patients with
isolated strains of the virus. Following criticism, the researchers maintained
that the children involved would receive better care than would otherwise
have been the case, and that strict conditions of parental consent had been
followed, including meticulous explanations in an environment of free choice.
Subsequent investigation and opinion, however, seriously challenged this.
Critics pointed to the fact that insufficient information for informed consent
was provided to parents, that those 'who consented' did not go on the waiting
list but were fast-tracked directly into the institution. Moreover, it is alleged
that the long-term risks were inadequately described and an insinuation

wrongly made that the children would receive a vaccine against the virus (Faden and Beauchamp, 1986; Kroll, 1993).[7]

Research abuses in social scientific settings

Even observational studies, a standard method in the social sciences and seemingly less invasive than those already mentioned, can carry significant risks. One famous case is usually referred to by the title of the book *Tea Room Trade*. In attempting to combat stereotyped attitudes towards homosexual men, Laud Humphreys posed as a 'watch queen' (to alert offenders to the approach of police) and observed hundreds of acts of fellatio in public restrooms. He gained the confidence of some of the people he observed and enlisted their aid in the study, but with numerous others he traced their addresses through licence plates and later, suitably disguised, deceptively interviewed them about their personal affairs.

Humphreys' work was important in that the findings cast doubt on numerous stereotypes, and his reply to numerous vociferous critics was that the importance of the research easily outweighed any violation of rights of privacy and self-determination. His critics argued that the moral wrong entailed by deception of this nature cannot be justified by appeals to beneficial consequences for society. No harm emanating from this study has been reported, but potential harm can arise in two ways. First, the harm from such studies can come from their intrusion alone, and, second, from error or abuse of confidentiality in the storing and communication of results.

Even in questionnaires and interviews where participation seems to be a completely voluntary matter, inquiry can be improper. In institutional settings in particular, subtle coercive forces often operate, and results obtained under the guise of anonymity can be intentionally or unintentionally misused, resulting in the exploitation of individuals. Seemingly innocuous questionnaires, such as teachers' attitudes towards classroom preparation, for example, could be misused for promotion purposes if strict anonymity is not maintained. This reinforces the view that when research is conducted utilising 'captive' populations, authority figures should not be involved in the research process at all, and should not have any access to data, as that would violate confidentiality requirements (Zelaznik, 1993). Moreover, the use of persons as gatekeepers who are higher up in an institution should never be thought to replace the informed consent of the participants themselves lest it be used as a vehicle to coerce those lower down the organisational ladder (Homan, 2002).

Milgram's research on obedience, first published in 1963, quickly assumed a position as a classic case study for problems of deception and consent. In studying obedience to authority his subjects were deceptively recruited and were not informed as to the actual methodology or objectives of the research. Put simply, the experiment proceeded as follows: the subject was required by the experimenter (authority figure) to administer electric shocks to a 'learner' (in reality an accomplice of the experimenter) as punishment for wrong answers in a learning process. The 'learner' only simulated pain, as no shocks were actually transmitted, a fact of which the subject was ignorant. When subjects expressed doubts about administering high voltage shocks, they were instructed by the experimenter to continue.

For many of the subjects, the experiment was an emotionally tense, traumatic experience, with at least one subject approaching nervous collapse at the prospect of the pain they were inflicting on the 'learners'. Subjects were debriefed, but critics condemned the research for the allegedly devastating psychological effects on some subjects, as well as for the deception practised and the lack of informed consent (Bok, 1978a; Faden and Beauchamp, 1986).

In a relevantly similar piece of research, in 1971 Philip Zimbardo conducted research in which paid student volunteers acted out the roles of prisoners and guards. The experiment was designed to examine the effects of a rigid institutional setting on attitudes and behaviour. Zimbardo prematurely terminated the experiment, as he observed that 'prisoners' were subjected to physical and psychological abuse by the 'guards', with the guards behaving in ways that brutalised and degraded their fellow research participants. He justified the study by contending that participants suffered no long-term negative consequences, and that the results assisted the process of prison reform. Nevertheless, his critics cited emotional stress, physical degradation, humiliation and the dubious utility of his results as problem areas.

While Zimbardo did obtain consent, which included disclosure of methodology and aims, it has been argued that it was abbreviated, inadequate and gave participants little indication of the stress that they would experience. The primary questions raised here are whether obtaining informed consent can justify very risky or scientifically questionable research, and whether one can consent to what is uncertain or unknown (Faden and Beauchamp, 1986).

Several problems, several solutions?

Both public and scientific opinion demanded responses to the research practices described above. Following the Second World War, 23 Nazi scientists involved in the 'biomedical' experiments described earlier were prosecuted; 16 of the doctors charged were found guilty.

The judgement at Nuremberg laid down a standard to which doctors had to conform when conducting experiments. This was the Nuremberg Code, and it can be considered the first major curb on research involving human subjects. It was intended to serve as a reference point for future research ethics codes, and an abbreviated version of its ten ethical and legal concepts is presented below:

1 The voluntary consent of the human subject is absolutely essential.
2 The experiment should be such as to yield fruitful results for the good of

society, unprocurable by other methods or means of study, and not random and unnecessary in nature.

3   The experiment should be so designed and based on the results of animal experimentation and a knowledge of natural history of the disease or other problem under study that the anticipated results will justify the performance of the experiment.

4   The experiment should be so conducted as to avoid all unnecessary physical and mental suffering and injury.

5   No experiment should be conducted where there is an *a priori* reason to believe that death or disabling injury will occur; except, perhaps, in those experiments where the experimental physicians also serve as subjects.

6   The degree of risk to be taken should never exceed that determined by the humanitarian importance of the problem to be solved by the experiment.

7   Proper preparations should be made and adequate facilities provided to protect the experimental subject against even remote possibilities of injury, disabilities or death.

8   The experiment should be conducted only by scientifically qualified persons. The highest degree of skill and care should be required through all stages of the experiment of those who conduct or engage in the experiment.

9   During the course of the experiment the human subject should be at liberty to bring the experiment to an end if he has reached the physical or mental state where continuation of the experiment seems to him to be impossible.

10 During the course of the experiment the scientist in charge must be prepared to terminate the experiment at any stage, if he has probable cause to believe, in the exercise of the good faith, superior skill and careful judgement required of him, that a continuation of the experiment is likely to result in injury, disability, or death to the experimental subject. (Kroll, 1993: 33–4)

Partly as a response to some of the questionable research described earlier, partly as an attempt to clarify, and in some case make practicable, the guidelines of the Nuremberg Code, and partly as a response to perceived threats to further biomedical research, the World Medical Association (WMA) began in the early 1960s to draft a more suitable code of research ethics.

The result was the Declaration of Helsinki in 1964, which, while enshrining the ideals of the Nuremberg Code, added the distinction of therapeutic versus non-therapeutic research, stipulating that 'the interest of science and society should never take precedence over considerations relative to the well-being of the subject' (Kroll, 1993: 34). The Declaration requires consent for all cases of non-therapeutic research, except where a subject is incompetent, in which case the support of a guardian is necessary.

Consent is not required in all cases of therapeutic research (Dawson, 2004),[8] and this is viewed by some as a weakness of the Declaration, particularly if a proposal passes through an inattentive review committee (Faden and Beauchamp, 1986). The Declaration has generated much debate, but at the very least it has served as a landmark or rallying point for subsequent codes of ethics, in that it served to further stimulate reflection and debate on the complex issues of informed consent and research ethics. It was a significant step by medical science towards self-regulation in that it was imposed internally, rather than externally as in the case of the Nuremberg Code. Finally, Helsinki and the codes it influenced provided evidence that the principles espoused in the Nuremberg Code should also apply to scientific investigations involving human subjects of a non-medical nature (Kroll, 1993).

Many sociologists have claimed that the biomedical model canonised in the Helsinki Declaration is inappropriately used as a template for social scientific research ethics (Homan, 1991). Bower and de Gasparis write:

> The regulation of human subject protection in social research seems not to have been stimulated by fears about the shenanigans of social scientists or the plight of their respondents, but rather to have been pulled along as an appendage to the regulations for the protection of biomedical research subjects who were seen to be at risk of quite tangible physical harm.
>
> (Bower and de Gasparis, 1978: 62)

While this may have the merits of aligning social research ethics as sequentially post-dating biomedical research ethics, it can also have the undesirable effect of inducing the thought that there is no significant problem in social scientific research (Diener and Crandall, 1978), which is an unjustifiable claim. Qualitative research in particular is addressed in detail in Chapter 7. Nevertheless, the case for the dominance of biomedical research and its framing effects in the ethics of social research can be made.

D'Agostino claims, more specifically, that the model has dominated for two separable reasons. First, in institutional terms it is biomedical ethics committees that have led the debate and policy development. Second, and more substantially, there are conceptual issues to be investigated. He writes:

> The aspects of the biomedical model which are embraced by most who work in this area are (i) its individual, local, and concrete orientation to questions about harm arising from scientific experimentation . . . and (ii) its stress on the device of informed consent in establishing the ethical probity of particular projects.
>
> (D'Agostino, 1995: 65)

This last remark is worth highlighting here. In particular, social scientists, have taken the claim to universality of informed consent to be a controversial colonising claim. They have argued (e.g. Homan, 1991, 2002) that some research may, indeed must, be carried out without the consent of the subjects or participants. They usually make reference to epistemological and ethical justifications. In the first instance it is argued that the very nature of human conduct means that to inform the subject of the precise nature of the research is to invalidate their responses. This is a well-known problem to psychological researchers and is discussed below (see Chapters 4 and 7). But this is often taken to be the first part of a justification – necessary but not sufficient. What most IRBs or RECs will require is an account of the value of such knowledge – its beneficence – in order to accept the method as ethically acceptable. An example of participant observation of soccer hooligans is one example that immediately springs to mind. These issues are further developed in Chapter 4.

The development of regulatory frameworks

The following years witnessed an escalation from the issuing of guidelines to the establishment of review procedures. In 1966 the NIH, the FDA and the DHEW started to issue detailed regulations to govern human subject research in medical and non-medical research supported by these agencies. In practice this meant that all recipients of NIH and Public Health Services (PHS) grants in the USA had to have had their research proposal approved by an ethics committee at their institution. This committee was responsible for considering the rights and welfare of subjects, the suitability of the methods used to obtain informed consent, and the potential risks and benefits of the research (Pettit, 1992).

In 1971 the DHEW issued its *International Guide to DHEW Policy on Protection of Human Subjects* (Liemohn, 1979), a detailed document that extended risk protocols to include possible psychological and social harm. There have been regular updates on this policy in the USA, with the latest Code of Federal Regulations of the Department of Health and Human Services being revised in June 2005 (DHHS, 2005). In 1974, the National Commission for the Protection of Human Subjects of Biomedical and Behavioural research was established, and contained a key provision charging Institutional Review Boards (IRBs) with reviewing research proposals involving human subjects. IRBs were thus now mandatory in institutions receiving federal grants.

Various regulations and interpretations have been recommended and adopted by many public and private organisations, extending policies of informed consent and protection of human subjects to any and all investigations. These include *inter alia* the American Alliance for Health, Physical Education, Recreation and Dance (AAHPERD), the American College of Sports Medicine, the American Psychological Association (APA), the British Association for Sport and Exercise Sciences (BASES), the British Sociological Association (BSA), the National Academy of Sciences, the Royal College of Physicians for all hospitals in England, as well as most major institutions of higher education (Kroll, 1993). In fact, particularly in the USA, the majority of universities have voluntarily adopted policies more restrictive than are required either by statute or by regulations as such (Pettit, 1992).

The response to research abuses has resulted in more intense scrutiny and regulation of research. Most research in exercise and sports science is conducted in universities, or in laboratories affiliated to universities. It is thus incumbent on researchers in such institutions (and elsewhere of course, such as national bodies, see for example the English Institute of Sport) to be aware of the ethical issues and responsibilities surrounding their work.

In the United Kingdom, the procedures for ethical approval of projects are neither as widespread nor as uniform as the regulations applied in the USA. Regional and local variations abound, and researchers must therefore check that they satisfy the requirements of their institution (e.g. university or laboratory), professional body (e.g. British Association of Sport and Exercise Sciences), the fund-granting agency (e.g. ESRC), and any other relevant authority (e.g. National Health Service Research Ethics Committee). Despite the historical lack of coordination, in the UK in particular, several recent initiatives have pushed research ethics and research governance to the forefront in the academic community. Just a few examples include the establishment of NHS Local Research Ethics Committees in the 1990s, the introduction into law of the European Clinical Trials Directive, and ESRC initiatives establishing a framework for research ethics in the social sciences.

It is often presumed by sceptics that those who know what is ethical will behave in moral ways, but this is not necessarily so. The regulations on medical ethics in Germany prior to the Second World War were detailed and stringent, yet they did not prevent abuses from occurring in prisoner-of-war camps, indicating that neither official endorsement nor high aspirations are enough to ensure protection for subjects. It is not just a historical problem either. Recently, one-third of Harvard University research projects were deemed ethically problematic by USA government investigators, and several research subject deaths have been reported, along with a host of other research ethics malpractices (Marcus, 2004: 14). Delineating the acceptable from the unacceptable in ethics in research involving human participants and subjects is not a settled issue. The principles we accept may be less conclusive, and the guidelines we apply may be less protective, than they appear to be (Capron, 1989). Constant review seems to be a prerequisite for research involving humans in exercise, health and sports.

2 What's in a name?

Ethics, ethical theories and research ethics

The variety of ethical inquiries

St Augustine famously asked 'What is time?' He answered by saying that if no one asked him then he knew, but if pushed for a definition he could not satisfactorily give an answer. He simply did not 'know'. It might seem to the reader that there exists a confusion of terms regarding morality, according to where they live and work. As will be discussed in Chapter 3, there is a terminological dispute as to whether the designations Research Ethics Committees (RECs) or Institutional Review Boards (IRBs) ought to be used. The former is typically used in the UK, while the latter is the dominant assignation in the USA. We note this to distinguish clearly what is merely a terminological dispute as opposed to a conceptual one. Sometimes, though, words commonly used as synonyms do harbour important conceptual distinctions. While we can, with little or no loss of meaning, substitute RECs and IRBs, we cannot simply exchange the words 'ethics' and 'morality' because of the complex conceptual disputes that these terms are merely a front for.

It is not unlikely that if one took a random selection of scientists and researchers who had just submitted a proposal for review by an REC, they would declare themselves in a similar position. Most would be able to cite examples of ethical and/or moral ideas in life as in research. A generic list might include items like 'duty', 'good character', 'obligation', 'principle', 'respect' or 'rights'. They might give instantiations of these ideas in research in terms of 'anonymity', 'consent', 'privacy' and so on. But, properly speaking, before we can understand at a more reflective level the scheme of things that allows us to recognise all the issues presented in Chapter 1, we must interrogate our understanding of the concepts of 'ethics' and 'morality'. This will entail, partly, some linguistic analysis and some stipulation. For there are as many definitions of these terms as there are theories spun from them.

One crude way of beginning might be to consider a range of paradigmatic cases of what people would call ethical or unethical in research. We know that making decisions involving issues such as harm, risks, benefits, confidentiality, data protection and so on are encountered in just about every research proposal, whether quantitative or qualitative or some combination of both. For example, in a physiology study, where a muscle biopsy may be required to answer a particular research question, a researcher needs to ask, *inter alia*, the following: will harm occur from the procedure; have adequate safety precautions been taken; have subjects been sufficiently informed regarding the procedures; have subjects freely consented to take part? In an ethnographic study, has one considered that a particular line of questioning may upset interviewees; do participants know that they can withdraw at any time without sanction; how will sensitive information be dealt with? These and many other questions impinge on the conduct and character of research, and researchers and lecturers themselves. Nevertheless, what might these disparate cases have in common such that we recognise them as ethical decisions or moral matters?

It may not surprise the reader to note that many philosophers, awkward beasts that they are, distinguish ethics from morality contrary to their ordinary meanings. It might be typical for Jane or John Smith to think that one's morality is what governs one's personal relations while ethics refers to more impersonal or institutional relations. In contrast, philosophers tend to reverse the meanings: 'ethics' is the local, particular, thick, stuff of personal attachments, projects and relations while 'morality', by contrast, is, detached, general (even universal), impartial, thin rules or norms governing how one should treat others or be treated by them. Typically, 'ethics' in this broad scheme of things, which – the reader will not be surprised to learn – is hotly contested, is prefigured by a the name of a particular group or institution: bioethics, business ethics, Christian ethics, feminist ethics, journalistic ethics, medical ethics, military ethics (if that is not an oxymoron), professional ethics, sports ethics and, of present concern, research ethics. This leaves us in something of a difficulty; how shall we understand ethics and research ethics in this book in a way that is coherent and defensible?

First, let us agree that ethics (at least for the purposes of this book) shall uncontroversially be taken to mean the philosophical study of morality. Yet what does 'the philosophical study of morality' mean? Well, many sociologists claim to be researching ethical issues in, say, ethnographies of football hooliganism, or dilemmas in nursing practice, or norms of authorship in laboratory-based experiments. These studies might entail gathering data first hand and critically commenting upon them. We are concerned with such studies only as a means to systematically reflecting upon them in order to evaluate *post hoc* whether the courses of action and the character of the research/ers are good, bad, defensible, indefensible or deplorable; or to consider the merits and defects of the design as would an REC in order to determine that such research is good. So our reflections will, in a clear way, be second order. We reflect on the good and the gruesome in research. But determining whether research falls under one heading and not the other, is not a straightforward matter. And the means by which we decide will betray the choices as to moral theory or the ethical position that we adopt. Even if we accept this designation of morality and ethics, there are still levels of ethics that it will be helpful to distinguish. In this chapter, we will distinguish three levels of ethics: (i) meta-ethics; (ii) normative ethics; and (iii) practical ethics. We shall say only a little about each of these levels. But a word of qualification is necessary here.

We are not suggesting that these levels are either given or necessary in any absolute way, nor that they are evaluatively naïve or theoretically innocent. The constructions of these levels of philosophical endeavour are a product of writings, over the centuries. And they are the product of Western philosophy. The extent to which other cultures might challenge the levels is not considered here. So, for example, many in the West have previously assumed that ethics are moral standards that apply to our general conduct as social beings, which are continuous with Christian moral teaching, such as adherence to the Ten Commandments. Different cultures have slightly different systems of thought. Yet in Africa, by contrast, the concept of Ubuntu regulates behaviour, and enjoins adherents to act to promote what might best be termed 'communal humanism'. We shall not reflect further on the challenges of cross-cultural norms or values in relation to levels of ethics, but instead address more pragmatically the issues these raise for researchers engaged in transcultural projects in Chapter 10.

It will be better to think of the levels of ethics, then, as a heuristic device; a way of managing the tortuous terrain of morality. We use them to help us think systematically about the issues of research design, data collection and analysis, report and scientific writing and so on. Neither we nor you, the reader, are logically compelled to think of ethics in this way. In attempting to ask the enduring philosophical questions – Why be moral? What are the strictures of morality? Which are the most pressing of morality's demands? Are moral demands universal? Is respect the cornerstone of morality? – these levels of ethics have been found useful.

Meta-ethics

Meta-ethics is that field of ethics where the philosophical abstraction is greatest. While moral philosophy generally attempts to deepen, revise and systematise reflection on how we believe we ought to conduct our lives, meta-ethics reaches to the foundational claims of all moral theories and practices. What are the grounds of moral authority? Is one moral theory more complete than any other? Can there be moral knowledge? Are moral principles unique in character? Are good and evil merely non-cognitive expressions of emotions or preferences? Do moral properties exist in the world or are they merely subjective or cultural constructs? These questions are among the most fundamental for all moral philosophers, sometimes called 'ethicists', to pursue.

Much deliberation in research ethics does not directly address these

questions and indeed simply assumes answers to do with the authority of
the beliefs of the IRB or REC as a legitimate organ of control, an institution-
ally justified gatekeeper for sound research. Most research ethics deliberation, by contrast, goes on at a very applied level, which oscillates between
normative and practical ethics.

Normative ethics

The impulse to systematise is among the most basic for philosophers.
Normative ethics shares with meta-ethics the need for abstraction from particular persons, or practices, or policies into clear, coherent and consistent
approaches. It might be useful to think that meta-ethics addresses issues that
relate in a foundational way to all moral theories. Normative ethics can then
be thought of as the development of moral theory or theories. There are
those who complain that if ethics is not practical then the philosophical
engine is somehow idling. While meta-ethics shapes the kind of moral
theory espoused, then normative ethics (theoretically informed moral positions) are in themselves a particular kind of theory. It has been argued
normative ethics should not to be thought of as a scientific theory (Williams,
1985) but rather as coherent and systematic reflection to guide our practices.
Some would argue that this thought properly belongs to meta-ethics. This
dispute illustrates nicely the difficulties of looking for hermetically sealed
categories in the levels of moral thought and practice. Uncontroversially, we
could say that normative ethics is thought to be substantive: it is about
getting one's hands dirty in the day-to-day stuff of life and offering at least
defensible solutions to practical problems of how we ought and ought not to
act. But it does so at a level that is consciously theoretically informed.

   In the sections that follow, we have identified five celebrated moral theories. Perhaps it is better to think of them as families of theories since they
each house a number of interpretations of a subtlety that we shall not
attempt to do justice to here. As with the levels of ethical reflection, it can be
helpful to distinguish two kinds of moral theories in a rather traditional way.
Some might be thought of as forward-looking, others backward-looking. We
do not mean to imply that some are traditional and others contemporary by
these vague labels. Rather, when confronted with a problem, we may attempt
to organise our reflections around things we hold important before the fact,
such as certain duties, obligations or rights. On the other hand we may look
to those things that will be directed towards the achievement of a certain
goal, such as the greatest benefit to a given population, or the achievement of
a desirable character trait such as honesty.

   In moral philosophy these two perspectives are usually given the label
deontology and teleology. In ancient Greek, *deontology* referred to the science
of duty (*deon* is taken to mean 'duty' roughly translated) while teleology
referred to the pursuit of a given purpose or goal (after *telos*). We will deal with
the theories under this description. We will first examine the deontological

family of theories (duty theory; rights theory) and then the teleological families (consequentialism – specifically utilitarian theory – and virtue theory). We will finally present what is probably the dominant approach in bioethics, principalism, an eclectic theoretical position which attempts to cater for deontological and teleological parameters of moral practice and thought.

Practical ethics

As the term implies, practical ethics is concerned with how we *ought* to act here and now. In the everyday contexts of research, academics find themselves asking such questions as: 'Am I obliged to present all data in my discussion or can I leave out certain factors that I deem irrelevant to the main thesis because they do not support it?', 'Can I break a promise of confidentiality if I think it will save a subject from being harmed wrongly or unnecessarily?', 'Ought I to accept research sponsorship from the tobacco or alcohol or even sports drinks industries?', 'Ought I to challenge sexist attitudes of interviewees if that will alter the data or harm the project irreparably?', 'Should I accede to including my supervisor's name on a project when I know that he has not contributed significantly towards the final article?', 'Are deceptive methods justifiable when researching the influence of drug sales representatives on doctors' prescribing habits?'

All these practical questions apply in everyday contexts in research. How we think about them will be informed or uninformed to the degree that we are willing to engage in philosophical reflections about their theoretical base. Whether we know it or not, indeed whether we care about it or not, our attitudes and choices with regard to the conflicts above will be nested within a set of theoretical considerations such as the duty to protect research subjects; the respect of colleagues; obligations to the profession; integrity to ourselves, and so on. What is being applied here is moral theory (knowingly or otherwise). The label 'practical ethics' is indeed relevant; we should not think that the term practical means non-theoretical. Rather it depicts a feature of morality that is widely accepted by philosophers: the conclusions of moral considerations should be action. Once we decide that a given problem is best considered in a given light, the conclusion that follows should be action-guiding. So practical or applied ethics should not be inert. An idea very much like this was propounded by Socrates over 2,400 years ago. It is captured in the phrase: 'Who knows the good chooses the good.' While philosophers have challenged the strong cognitivist line (that simply knowing what to do will somehow transport us directly to act) from a variety of lines of argument (notably Aristotle argued for the existence of the possibility of weakness of will in the face of knowing what we must do), we still argue that as a general norm knowing what ought to be done in research contexts places researchers under a certain ethical pull toward doing the right thing, and being a good person not merely a technically effective researcher.

An awareness of central philosophical theories should, in principle, serve us well in research situations where we begin to understand the push and pull of competing courses of thought, feeling and action. An awareness of such theories can certainly help towards coherent, consistent and transparent modes of response. In short, it can make responses both accountable and transparent. We shall develop these ideas specifically in the context of research ethics below.

First, we shall consider some summary outlines of consequence-based, duty-based, rights-based and virtue-based moral theories more generally. Again, it should be noted by way of caveat that each of these sketches represents not one theory but a whole family of theories under these labels. Several excellent collections now exist for the reader who wishes to familiarise themselves with these families of theories, and the wreckages of many others that are to be found at the bottom of the moral philosophical ocean (see, for example, Singer, 1993; Lafollette, 2000). We have selected duty, rights and consequentialist theories since they represent the dominant modern moral theories, and we also comment on the ancient virtue-based ethics since the last quarter of a century has seen a very significant revival of interest in it.

Consequentialism

The idea that religion unequivocally provided us with moral rules justified a picture of a kind of moral law. What drove human beings to act rightly was observance of its authority. Consequentialism, by contrast, appeals to the empirical, the here and now of human welfare. It is driven by the idea that what human beings seek is that which is good for them and that they seek to avoid what is not of benefit to them. In a famous passage, the founder Jeremy Bentham claimed that pleasure and pain were our sovereign masters. It followed then that questions of moral rightness or wrongness hinge upon assessment of good (pleasurable) and bad (painful) consequences. At first sight, ethically evaluating research would seem a perfectly natural extension of utilitarian thinking. What we first look for in research is very often related to the question of what benefits it will bring and what drawbacks too. This is nothing if not consequentialist thinking.

Perhaps the most well-known form of consequentialism is utilitarianism associated most famously with John Stuart Mill, and his book *Utilitarianism* first published in 1861. It is the clearest exposition of the theory first developed by Jeremy Bentham (see his *An Introduction to the Principles of Morals and Legislation*, first published in 1789).

The basic idea in this moral theory is quite simple, and is captured in this passage from Mill:

> actions are right in proportion as they tend to promote happiness, wrong as they tend to promote the reverse of happiness. By happiness is meant

pleasure and the absence of pain; by unhappiness, pain and the privation of pleasure.

(Mill, 1962 [1863]: 257)

Utilitarianism claims that morality is concerned with doing good, so that when we assess the morality of what we choose to do our only consideration should be the utility of acting in one way or another. 'Utility' or 'good' can have a number of meanings including pleasure, happiness, welfare and the satisfaction of preferences. All of these conceptualisations can be considered under the heading 'beneficence' – a principle of action aimed toward good. Equally, when considering the goodness of certain outcomes we must also consider potential harmful consequences in the form of pain, or general disbenefit. These are generally captured under the principled heading non-maleficence: though strictly speaking this refers to non-harm and is a cornerstone of medical ethics. The Latin phrase *primum non nocere* (first do no harm) captures this principle most famously. But this might be a principle adopted by deontologists as we shall see below.

Utilitarianism is therefore commonly described as an 'outcome morality': when evaluating or attempting to justify a course of action, utilitarians weigh up potential outcomes of each possibility based on the premise that what ought to be done is always whatever produces greater utility. This is often referred to, after Jeremy Bentham, as the Greatest Happiness Principle.

A chief value of the utilitarian approach is that it provides a method for noting and evaluating benefits and harms even if it is not quite the precise mathematical morality its founders envisaged. Utilitarianism is based on Bentham's 'felicific calculus' which is essentially a means of rational calculation by such measures as the intensity, certainty, extent, nearness in time and duration of pleasure or happiness attained by a given policy or action. A major appeal of utilitarianism, then, is that it produces a right answer in any given situation according to the criteria above. All manner of difficult choices are grouped together and solved merely by seeking a balance between competing considerations that promises to produce the best outcome. However, there are a number of problems with the 'felicific calculus' as we shall see.

A further point must be made in praise of utilitarianism, which relates to philosophical and common-sense language. When the term 'utilitarian' is used in everyday contexts it is often as a term of abuse. Thus, describing a researcher's attitude as 'utilitarian' means little more than that conveying the opinion that the researcher merely used their participant as a means to his or her own ends, subject to their will as researcher. By contrast, the philosophical theory 'utilitarianism' has at its core an impartial ethic. Anyone relevantly affected by a course of action should be counted in terms of harms and benefits. Researchers, or the group they belonged to, could never privilege themselves in the calculation. So to describe the Nazi researchers of our previous chapters as 'utilitarian' would clearly be to invoke the rather general meaning the term has acquired and should not be seen as a proper philosophical designation of the term.

It is necessary also to distinguish between act and rule utilitarianism. The former invokes a utilitarian application in relation to this or that given act whereas the latter considers the consequences if the given action were to be considered as a typical course of action. A given course of action, say in disclosing the identity of a research participant, may yield greater benefits than observing the standard condition of privacy or anonymity. But what if this were to lead to a situation where revealing the identity of participants became more widespread? Under such a consideration act-utilitarianism looks short-sighted and yields in the medium or long term more harm than good.

One of the appealing features of utilitarianism is that it provides a common *currency* of moral action and justification wherein competing courses of action can be evaluated in terms of a single measure (Williams, 1972). This procedure is *prima facie* appropriate for the evaluation of research, as, with the increasing emphasis on efficiency, effectiveness, and financial accountability, utilitarianism provides a workable framework of evaluation. It allows in our considerations all benefits of the research to be counted and compared. It might allow the evaluator to entertain efficiency considerations. If the same outcomes can be reached by less expenditure, cheaper methods, or equally if the proposed research already duplicated existing research, we would be able to come to a clear decision as to its benefits or disbenefits. There are, however, considerable difficulties in comparing and calculating alternatives.

One problem for researchers concerns the pain or pleasure that is attached to the research. Although Bentham (1948) believed that happiness was a mental state, that someone is happy when in a state of pleasure and no pain, it is not always easy to interpret or apply this to actual research cases. Compare the added gain in precise data from taking gases to evaluate lactate production in the body with muscle biopsy. The former is not invasive – though perhaps a little uncomfortable to the participant on the treadmill. Biopsies, by contrast, require the insertion of a fairly large needle into the belly of the muscle and withdrawal such that a portion of the muscle is extricated for analysis. Utilitarians would, in principle, be able to evaluate the harm to a small number of participants against the potentially large benefit to the scientific and athletic communities (athletes, coaches).

But is it true that we can really compare these benefits and harms? Would it not vary according to how each participant experienced the biopsy – well or badly carried out? Is it true that we can make these interpersonal comparisons or additions? Would the enforced rest have the same consequences for each of the participants? How would we 'count' the scientific value of gaining more precise data? How would we know whether repeating the same experiment with different control groups really gave us a gain in scientific knowledge? This basic example highlights important weaknesses of utilitarianism considered as a simple summing of benefit and harms to evaluate research by. Ultimately, too much time and effort may be spent in trying to identify the infinite consequences and complications of potential utilitarian calculations of actions. The *reductio ad absurdum* of such a position is a life of calculating. As Solomon (1993: 256) puts it, 'pending investigation' may be the only moral course of (for example) IRB/REC members in such situations.

Duty-based (deontological) moral theory

The idea of a moral theory developed as a moral law is typically attributed to the German philosopher Immanuel Kant and is set out in his *Groundwork of the Metaphysic of Morals*, first published in 1785. His was a moral law of universal duties. Despite its modern provenance, the term itself belongs to ancient Greece. It is the coupling of two words *deon* (duty) and *logos* ('reason' or 'science', very roughly translated). On this theory, moral rightness involves acting out of respect for moral duty. Further, according to this position, one should act out of respect for moral duty regardless of the consequences of so doing. So, promoting the welfare of research participants would not be a concern to the deontologist strictly speaking. What matters most is doing one's moral duty, irrespective of the consequences.

Given that doing one's duty is the cornerstone of deontology, one critical question that ought to be raised by this approach is precisely how one determines what one's duty is.

It should be noted that the 'Categorical Imperative' that Kant took to be the cornerstone of his moral system, requires a little elaboration since there is not one interpretation but two. In the first instance, by wedding morality and rationality, Kant sets out what is to count as a moral rule. All moral rules, he argued, must be such that we would will *all* persons to act in accordance with them. In everyday language this is the 'do as you would be done to' rule. It seeks to universalise our thought and action so that we never privilege ourselves or our favoured ones; it thus underwrites and reinforces the notion of moral impartiality which one of the cornerstone of utilitarian moral philosophers thinking and their social reform programme. The second interpretation of the 'Categorical Imperative' urges us never to treat other people as means to our ends, but rather as ends in themselves, since all human agents are worthy of our unconditional respect, because they are moral agents.[1] It is clear that both notions operate in the ethical evaluation of research.

Consider the issue of deception in research (which we shall discuss more fully in Chapters 4 and 7). Ought we to approve of deceptive methods in a given research design? Kant's answer, roughly, is that one should ask whether one could approve of everyone acting in the same way in which one intends to act. So if one is considering deceiving participants, Kant's line is that one puts to oneself the question: 'Could I approve of everyone acting as I intend to now?' If one could, then one has acted out respect for moral duty. (Other possible sources of duty include the law, moral intuition and God.) If one could not then the contrary was indicated. In some cases this rather thin, blanket rule is applied without careful consideration of the description of the act. Would one consider telling one's partner a white lie to remove them from the house in order to set up a surprise birthday party an act of deception? More obviously, however, it is the second of the interpretations of the Categorical Imperative that has exercised research ethicists. Clearly the outstanding examples of this that we have outlined in Chapter 1 above fall under the very general description of research and researchers who have used other human beings[2] merely as a means to the ends of the researchers, the political system or wider social institutions.

In support of this kind of moral theory, it may be there are some kinds of acts that are simply wrong and can never be justified, e.g. killing an innocent child. For the utilitarian, if harming one research participant or subject would lead to more overall utility it could be morally justified. Duty-based moral theory captures the intuition that some things are absolutely wrong, some moral duties absolutely compelling, e.g. not to steal, not to kill the innocent, not to lie and so on. Moreover, as we shall see below (pp. 41–3), deontological ideas such as the respect for autonomy feature very heavily in the Four Principles approach to applied ethics that is dominant in the health and medical spheres of research ethics.

Rights-based theory

Many doctors are aware of the way in which detainees, patients and prisoners were dealt with during the Second World War. As already described, the outrage that followed gave birth to the Nuremberg Code, and later the Helsinki Declaration, which were designed to specify the rights that persons could expect *inter alia* from the medical and healthcare professions. The rights that ensued are widely thought to be universally enjoyed by humans in virtue of their humanity. We now take for granted in the West the existence and self-evidency of certain rights: to free speech, free association and movement. We also take for granted that these are powers enjoyed by individuals rather than larger social groups such as families or communities.

The term 'right(s)', however, is not straightforward to understand. Although the term is naturally associated with the law, moral rights are not co-extensive with legal ones. Of course the extension of rights claims to foetuses and non-human animals, which also have interests, has been a matter of considerable controversy. The issue of the use of non-human animals in research has been a highly charged one both legally and politically. It is, however, beyond the scope of this book. For our purposes we can think of rights as claims or powers either to promote or protect the interests of research participants but also researchers themselves (see Waldron, 1989; Almond, 1993). Such rights are often taken as absolute or inviolable. Typically, the invocation of rights is designed to protect the moral boundaries of a person against other considerations such as economy, efficiency or political or financial expediency.

The notions of rights and duties are commonly coupled. If a participant has a right to know the nature and scope of the research they will be a part of there appears to be, other things being equal, a duty upon researchers to inform her or him. In the case of minors this can becomes problematic. We discuss the issue of vulnerable research participants in Chapter 10. We may first need to determine who enjoys the right: parent or participant – and in some cases researcher or participant. The idea that a rights-based approach might exhaustively cater for research ethics has never, to our knowledge, been seriously mooted. While it is not claimed by anyone to be sufficient, however, there are few ethicists who would ever claim that the claims it makes – often with close relatives in legal rights enjoyed by participants, researchers and subjects alike – can be ignored. Claiming properly that one's interests ought to be promoted or protected within research is indeed a powerful tool in the governance of research.

Virtue-based (aretaic) theory and feminist ethics

Virtue-based theories are described as aretaic since their exposition is often traced back to the Ancient Greeks for whom virtue, or excellence of character, is translated as *aréte*. Aristotle is often taken as the great virtue theorist. His ethics were founded on practical wisdom supported by a well-disposed and settled set of personality traits which are typically called virtues. In recent times virtue theory has enjoyed something of a renaissance (see MacIntyre, 1986; Blum, 1993) while feminist ethics has a much more recent history (see Baier, 1993; Tronto, 1993).

While the foregoing theories concentrate principles of action – what we ought to do in order to act morally – the currency of virtue ethics is the character of the person or human agent. As we have seen, the course of action is typically driven by some principle or rule to protect or promote rights, respect duty or maximise welfare. For virtue theorists, however, the central question, which is prior to the moral problems or dilemmas that one faces, is rather of the kind 'How ought I to live my life?' or 'What kind of person am I to be?' or 'What would my chosen role-model feel, think, and do?'

A common moral intuition, and one supported by many modern moral theories, is the idea of universality. All persons deserve to be treated equally. In contrast to this, virtue ethics is often described as particularist or situationist. The virtue theorist is not strongly guided by principles but allows the particular features of a situation to play a determining role in what it is best to do and be. This gives virtue theory an adverbial quality: we admire in, and expect from, medical professionals such traits as 'honesty', 'integrity', 'responsibility', 'truthfulness' and so on. Even if one acknowledges rights or duties that apply in a given situation, only a person of good character assures praiseworthy action and the avoidance of culpable choices.

Feminist ethics are often thought of as a species of virtue ethics. Unlike the impartiality and objectivist spirit of modern moral theories (deontology, rights, utilitarianism), feminist ethics makes primary the notion of connectedness of human agents. This gives a special place in its ethical thought to virtues that display best the concern for human connectedness such as 'care', 'compassion' or 'trust'. In contrast to what it conceives of as the cold and quasi-scientific impartialism of modern moralities (Gilligan, 1982) it actively promotes the interests and welfare of women and girls. In the context of research, a focus on women's issues, enacted by female researchers, often embodies an overtly democratic set of aims intended to further female interests in the design and promotion of the research.

This leaves virtue theorists and feminist ethicists open to a charge of over-flexibility or inconsistency. How do we know which virtues ought to be elicited by which situations and persons therein? Moreover, is it true that different societies in different epochs have valued different kinds of traits? Virtue theory, it is said, under-determines right action and engenders inconsistent or unequal approaches. It gives little guidance, it is said, to the researcher who wonders should they be honest with the injured athlete's employers or compassionate with respect to their athlete as participant?

A note about intuitionism, subjectivism and relativism

It is often held that, when deciding upon courses of action, and finding oneself in a quandary, the only recourse is to one's intuition. Clearly, it is thought, there are no facts to settle the matter, there will always be some unreasonable clash of opinions, so the sole court of appeal is to the working of one's heart and mind (so to speak). It could be said that the foregoing theories were designed precisely to rule out the kind of inconsistency or (worse) simple capriciousness, which the resort to intuitionism is thought to entail. Principally, the appeal to one's intuitions is thought to be problematic since one's intuitions are a hostage to all manner of bias based upon one's upbringing, class, educational background and so on. So the intuition of one may be another's worst nightmare and vice versa. Equally, there would be no check on the consistency of one's intuitions from one day to the next, or on any given issue. Inconsistency, contradiction and worse are endorsed (it is said) by appeal to mere intuitions. This is not to say that one's intuitions are necessarily awry but rather that, alone, they offer an all-too-fallible guide to doing the right things and being the right kind of person.

In discussions of what is acceptable and unacceptable, right or wrong, in research one often hears the labels 'subjectivism' or 'relativism' – especially when differences of view emerge. They are often used as a way of preserving one's own (righteous?) position in the face of opposition. Often they are little more than an egoistic clinging to one's own preferred position to which one has failed to give critical self-scrutiny. Equally they are often used as stoppers – a way of disengaging in argument and discourse:

thus, 'It's all a matter of opinion' is the commonest subjectivist exhortation. For the relativist, the popular refrain is that X or Y is simply foisting the norms of their group onto others, which is to commit the gravest postmodern sin.

In any of the three theories outlined above, a person is typically thought to behave immorally when they act selfishly without regard for harms to others. Researchers who merely use their subject pool as fodder for their (supposedly) all-important research are exemplifying subjectivity in their lack of consideration. Some very clear examples exist in the history of psychological research, and also early sports science research, where lecturers simply used novice students as a data pool as part of their studies – without ever properly offering informed consent. We discuss this particular issue in Chapter 8. But, for present purposes, it is worth dwelling a little on the ideas of objectivity, subjectivity and relativism. To be sure these issues belong to meta-ethics, but they do surface frequently in discussions over whether one should approve a certain research project and even in the development of particular methodologies. To describe a particular research programme or interpretation as subjective is usually to dismiss it as unscientific. It refers to the fact that the authority of a particular judgement or position is the person (i.e. the subject) him or herself. There is another sense of 'subjective' in philosophical parlance, which is the equivalent of relativism. Sociologists typically reserve the term 'relativism' for cultural rather than individual application (cultural relativism), where it means that standards of rightness are not universal but rather relative *inter alia* to a particular time, place, age, gender, culture or society. Here the contrast is with the idea of a universal objectivity – often referred to as absolutism – that moral standards apply to all persons in all times and places. This position is anathema for anthropologists and sociologists alike (see Sugden, 2002, 2005). Now, although absolutism is a radical position (sometimes held by religiously inspired ethics), it is important to stress the idea that subjectivism at the individual level is no more acceptable than relativism at the social level. Neither supplies any *critical* guide to conduct. In the first case, whatever is right is so because I say it. In the second, whatever is right is simply the case because it is the dominant norm (at the moment, in this place, at this time, with respect to these contexts and so on). Neither offers a critical and enduring guide to action – yet we know that professional regulations with respect to research exist principally as a foil to both subjectivism and relativism.

Principled theories and composite principled ethics

It is important to note that the three theoretical positions sketched above do share some important resemblances. It is typically said that they are each impartial, universally binding and prescriptive (or action-guiding). The precise ways in which the theories are thought to be action-guiding is itself interesting to note. We shall discuss the ways in which theories and cases relate to each other shortly. For the moment we observe that each theory aims toward settling a course of conduct in a manner that is 'objective' as opposed to 'subjective', both in the sense of being egoistic and/or unprincipled.

In the field of bioethics, the idea of a principled ethic has achieved widespread use and, perhaps it is fair to say, a certain dominance. It is not sufficient simply to describe or label this approach as a 'principles' approach (as it is sometimes referred to by way of shorthand) since we can think of each of the theories above as principled. In utilitarianism the principle is of maximising good consequences. In deontology the guiding principle is that of one's duty. In rights theory the guiding principle is that of protecting and promoting the interests of persons. Each is principled then, it is just that the principles each theory espouses do not necessarily cohere, and very often appear to clash.

The most famous and widely applied composite principled approach in applied ethics emerged largely as a response to publicly aired conflicts and problems in medicine during the 1960s and 1970s in North America. The response was formulated in *The Belmont Report* and is given its most sophisticated expression in Beauchamp and Childress's text *Principles of Biomedical Ethics*. While it emerged in 1978 it is now in its fifth edition and it has evolved in response to rigorous and often vehement criticism of its approach. Beauchamp and Childress developed an approach to ethical reasoning and decision-making comprising four moral principles that can be brought to bear on moral problems in medicine – though clearly they might be thought, at least on the face of it, to apply to all health research too. The basic principles operate as a framework rather than a method (Beauchamp and Childress, 2001; Gillon, 2003). Indeed they talk of clusters or principles, which serve as guidelines for professional ethics:

1   *respect for autonomy* (a norm of respecting the decision-making capacities of autonomous persons);
2   *nonmaleficence* (a norm of avoiding the causation of harm);
3   *beneficence* (a group of norms for providing benefits and balancing benefits against risks and costs); and
4   *justice* (a group of norms for distributing benefits, risks and costs fairly).
                                        (Beauchamp and Childress, 2001: 12)

They argue that these basic principles are to be found in most classical ethical theories. We have seen above how respect for autonomy is central to deontological ethics,[3] and how that theory might serve to uphold non-maleficence, while it is clear that utilitarianism is centrally concerned with beneficence. Nevertheless, utilitarianism has historically been criticised for being rather unconcerned with justice at the expense of the greater good, while deontology has typically been thought silent on issues of balancing benefit and harm. The principle of justice might be thought central to issues of respect in deontology. There is surely some strong justification for Beauchamp and Childress's claim that their basic principles are well chosen.

What is often, but loosely, referred to as the medical model of research is frequently followed in exercise physiology research without thought with regard to its application, the supposition being that if it is the standard for the medical profession it is surely appropriate for us. Yet not only is there a critical debate as to whether the model of medical research ethics is applicable to all forms of medical research, the idea of extending it to all research in exercise, health and sports generates yet further problems about its applicability. We take up this contrast in various sections of the book, but especially in Chapter 4, on informed consent.

Ethical theories and research ethics

As researchers we may be given guidance as to how to make ethical decisions in respect of the formulation of our research aims or goals and of course the means or methods to achieve them. We may be given feedback on our proposals by colleagues and supervisors, or more formally through the ethics review process. In addition to such guidance as we might receive, however, it is still incumbent on all researchers, as responsible human agents, personally and carefully to consider the ethical issues involved in our projects, and to make considered judgements in the light of the ethical theories presented.

Having offered a sketch of ethical theories above, and reasons as to why they are preferable to positions such as intuitionism, relativism or subjectivism, it is now necessary to move from general to more specific ethical questions. As researchers or aspirant researchers, we will be faced with particular and sometimes unique moral questions. The question will no longer be 'What ought I do?' but 'What ought I do in this instance?' This means that we will be confronted by situationally specific ethical issues, and we will need to *apply* ethical judgements so that we can proceed with appropriate actions. Is it possible, however, to usefully employ moral theory to help us penetrate the complexity of the human situation to generate a rationally consistent response to real-world ethical problems?

Throughout the world, departments of philosophy are now offering courses in medical ethics, research ethics, environmental ethics, business and professional ethics and so on. Similarly, research methods courses in health sciences or sports and exercise sciences (or any of the numerous degrees in the field that fall under similar names) invariably have a research ethics component. Why is this so? One important reason for the growth of applied ethics is that it is a response to new problems resulting from developing technology. For example, advances in medicine have raised perplexing questions about the definition of death, questions that need to be answered when applied to practical situations of organ transplantation. With regard to sport, questions of personhood and natural states need to be considered when looking at performance-enhancing substances. Further, in exercise and health scientific research, invasive interventions and procedures are increasingly adopted, whether physical (as with muscle biopsies or blood-taking) or mental (as in psychological interventions).

To advocate a 'hands-off' approach to normative issues arising in research would constitute not only an abnegation of the traditional goal of moral philosophy (i.e. of understanding the nature of the good life), but also an unacceptable disengagement from important moral issues. The disengagement of scientists should be thought of as culpable. The issues of research ethics abuse set out in the last chapter require the sort of insight that philosophical thinking is able to provide (Borchert and Stewart, 1986). This is supported by Veatch (1989), who holds that there is no reason to assume that being skilled in, for example, medical science, will make one expert in choosing among conflicting courses of actions.

We ought also to inquire, though, why we should not also hold philosophers who work in these spheres to account. We argue throughout the text that philosophers ought properly to engage with researchers from other disciplines so that the conduct of research may be enhanced. Such engagement is driven, with eloquence, by the promptings of the feminist ethicist Baier who writes:

> Can we approve of a division of labor in which the theorists keep their hands clean of real-world applications, and the ones who advise the decision makers, those who do 'applied ethics', are like a consumer reports service, pointing out the variety of available theories and what costs and benefits each has for a serious user of it? Does the profession of moral philosophy now display that degeneration of a Kantian moral outlook that Hegel portrays, where there are beautiful souls doing their theoretical thing and averting their eyes from what is happening in the real world, even from what is happening in the way of 'application' of their own theories, and there are those who are paid to be the 'conscience' of the medical, business or legal profession, what Hegel calls the moral *valets*, the professional moral judges?
>
> (Baier, 1985: 236)

Applying ethics to research ethics scenarios

In summary, we might think that knowledge of basic philosophical and ethical positions is highly valuable in thinking through the thickets of research ethics, but are we able to articulate what that value consists in? To decide to pursue a certain course of action is to decide that it is more defensible or less harmful than available alternatives, and this inescapably means making value judgements. Making these judgements may involve making ethical choices. Some of these choices may be made instinctively, but in other cases our intuitions may fail us, or they may conflict with the intuitions or convictions of other people. In any event, as we have noted above, intuition is not a reliable arbiter of moral judgement. When making ethical choices, the process would ideally involve disciplined, rigorous and systematic reflection on intuitions, convictions and facts before making a considered judgement as to what is morally right or wrong, praiseworthy or blameworthy, empathic or egoistic. An awareness of philosophy in thinking through issues of research ethics will emphasise the application of analytical skill and attempt to prevent the overriding influence of purely personal attitudes, prejudices or intuitions in making moral judgements.

One particular difficulty, then, for members of research ethics committees, or supervisors, or indeed researchers with some familiarity with ethical theories, lies in pinning down the precise manner of applying the theories. Moreover, it could be contended that the fundamental principles, whether deontological or utilitarian, commonly regarded as constituting the core of ethical theory are too general and vague to apply determinately to concrete, real situations. It could be said also that applying rights will not settle many of the various research ethics quandaries. Equally, merely exhorting researchers to be virtuous might be said to be less than helpful when one is not clear which virtue should trump which in a given situation. The question that arises is whether, and if so how, these central ethical concepts are to be brought to bear on a particular problem.

The complexity of cases in, for example, research ethics may allow reasonable people to apply the same principle in different ways, or different principles in the same situation. The substantive moral work occurs in determining how a principle, norm or character trait might impinge upon a particular problem, but the resources for addressing that issue are external to the principles themselves. So, on this view, conceptual analysis can make only a limited, albeit important, contribution to practical morality, and 'although conceptual analysis can elevate a concept from the status of being "radically confused" to the status of being "essentially contested", it cannot go on to resolve the dispute in which that concept figures' (Hoffmaster, 1992: 1423).

This of course all serves to question the applicability of ethical concepts in various situations. Autonomy, for example, is considered to be the most central of ethical concepts in research ethics, yet it is necessary to consider which meaning or dimension of autonomy is being adverted to. We can distinguish four separate, though related, senses of the concept of 'autonomy' that may apply: autonomy as free action; autonomy as authenticity, autonomy as effective deliberation, and autonomy as moral reflection. Which sense should apply in particular situations? What if some of these conflict in specific cases?

The answer to questions such as these must turn on an assessment of underlying substantive considerations, not further refinement of the concept of autonomy (Hoffmaster, 1992). A further difficulty is that although a multiplicity of ethical considerations may be said to apply to moral problems in a particular field, when two or more of these conflict, as they often do, there often appears no way of resolving the conflict. Simply conceiving research ethics as applied ethics give us no hierarchical ordering of principles, and no procedure for comparing their merits. As a last resort, people often invoke general ethical theories, e.g. deontology or utilitarianism, but the same difficulty emerges at this level, namely, conflict arises and the theory has no mechanism to resolve it.

Research ethics as casuistry?

The above is a criticism of research ethics as a theory-driven approach. Rachels once described it as the 'straightforward application model' (2001: 15). Ethics in real-life settings cannot simply be a case of adding theory to situation and computing the ethical solution with the help of moral philosophical theory. Rather, it is said by some that we should conceive of the thrust of research ethics from the precisely opposing direction; not from theory to practice, from the general to the particular, but rather from the particular to the general. Particular situations are as always situated in social, cultural, and historical milieux. Hoffmaster captures this sensibility particularly well:

> actual moral decision-making is situational – it is tailored to the demands of particular circumstances as well as the capacities and limitations of the persons enmeshed in those circumstances.
>
> (Hoffmaster, 1992: 1425)

Some will feel that acknowledging the particularity of situations is flirting with relativism. Those strongly committed to any of the theories above, or indeed the four principles approach, will use the term 'casuistry' to characterise this approach. In calling a line of reasoning 'casuistic' they will intend a term of abuse to the reasoner. Nevertheless, there are arguments in favour of understanding of researchers attempting to construe ethical issues in research in a contextually or situationally sensitive way. Casuists will typically reason for the rightness or desirability of a given course of action (or its converse) by way of analogy, or by appealing to previous precedents with relevantly similar particulars (Jonsen and Toulmin, 1988). As Arras (2001) notes, this way of working lacks the parsimony and elegance that are taken to be the hallmarks of scientific theory and moral theory alike. It is precisely this anti-scientific picture of ethics that the celebrated British philosopher Bernard Williams (1985) spoke of when he remarked that whatever kind of theory ethics could yield, it could not be like that of a scientific theory. Its history lies in the ancient art of rhetoric. This method is much more likely, Arras (2001) argues, to appeal to a wider public because it will not have alienated those who object to the preferred foundational principle: respect, rights, or utility. He writes:

> This kind of multifaceted rhetorical appeal typically yields moral conclusions that are admittedly apodictic; but the casuist argues, again

following Aristotle, that this is the best we can hope for when arguing about particulars.

(Arras, 2001: 110)

We contend, thus, that a casuistic approach is the best approach to characterise consideration of research ethics. Consensus can be reached without digging down to foundational principles that not uncommonly clash. In pluralistic settings it can allow a plurality of considerations and voices without developing a practical mêlée or indeed a theoretical impasse. It is of course open to external critique. By looking back to precedent or paradigm, it could be argued that it has not the resources to cope with new scenarios. It could also be argued that a certain amount of conservativism or, worse, uncritical acceptance of the status quo, adheres to casuistry in its appeal to previous cases. This objection cannot be fully refuted. Yet, if we accept that all approaches are open to critique, it may well be that a casuistic approach, which begins from particulars and moves out to the general considerations of research ethics – found in codes of conduct, committees' rulings, and institutional guidance – is the best we can hope for.

Accepting a casuistic approach does not mean that we necessarily place our judgements and rulings on a slippery slope to relativism. It simply means that we prioritise the importance of individual circumstances and their particularity, that we accept that principles and norms may have different weightings in different situations, and that we acknowledge that codes of conduct may have guidelines that are inappropriate in certain cases.

Conclusion: the limits of ethics in research

Does the rise in recent decades of research ethics within research methods courses and university governance systems mean that researchers and research ethics committees will reach definitive answers to thorny ethical questions, and does it mean that human subject abuse will cease? The answer is 'No' on both counts. In the application of ethics, it seems that there is an expectation that final and transcendent resolution of ethical disputes is possible. However, ethical systems do not exist in order to eliminate ethical discourse. Rather, they provide a working framework for such discourse – a framework for the confrontation of particular situations that pose ethical problems.

In short, the practice of philosophical ethics provides mechanisms for critically reasoned and systematic approaches to our problems in research. It does not aim necessarily at finality. In an affirmative answer to the second question above, it could perhaps be argued that a repeat of past human subject abuses is unlikely in today's moral climate. However, acceptance of such an argument should be approached with caution. Given the nature of research and the 'progress imperative' of sciences in general, it is hardly surprising that society continues to allow and encourage human experimentation. In this scenario, it has become evident that legislation is not sufficient to curb excesses where information is demanded.

In research methods courses, students are typically told that 'the ethical issues need to be considered as part of research'. Yet precisely what is meant by this, and what the relations between research and ethics might be, is seldom made clear. We have tried to show how these terms are contested within a range of families of theories. We have argued that such theories are necessary to combat subjectivism or relativism in our review of the ethics of research. It may be sufficient to rest at this: as researchers or members of research ethics committees, we want our judgements not merely to be acceptable but to be coherent, consistent and, if not praiseworthy then certainly above reproach or blame.[4] This necessitates the adoption of reason in systematically thinking through the harms and benefits of research both in terms of the desired goals and the methods and processes to achieve them. The clearest way of doing this is to consider our moral decisions within a framework of established ethical theories, though not slavishly applying one at the expense of others. We prescribe no *particular* method or theory here. We are content merely to point to the existence of certain widely followed ethical theories and how these can inform, in a casuistical way, the decisions of researchers and research ethics committees in coming to ethically defensible judgements and actions. Now of course it might be argued that the adoption of a casuistical approach is itself 'theory-laden' or at least not theoretically innocent. If all that is meant by this is the disavowal of deductively applied moral positions then we plead guilty as charged.

3   Research governance

The ethics review and approval processes

The emergence of research governance

Research in exercise, health and sports sciences, even more than other forms of investigation involving human participants, has experienced rapid growth over the last three or four decades. As we noted in Chapter 1, in biomedical and behavioural research, past abuses and scandals resulted in legislative and regulatory responses such as the Nuremberg Code and the Helsinki Declaration. Subsequent to this, Institutional Review Boards (IRBs) or Research Ethics Committees (RECs),[1] were formed on a widespread basis. These developments changed the face of research by requiring researchers to justify the goals and methods of their research on/with humans to peer investigators and to review group procedures prior to recruiting participants (Annas, 1991).

The general heading under which these issues fall is 'research governance'. What this means, however, is not universally agreed. One recent offering is sufficiently clear to indicate the terrain. Shaw *et al.* (2005: 497) define research governance as 'the system of administration and supervision through which research is managed, participants and staff are protected, and accountability is assured'. They go on to note, like many others, that precisely how this idea is effected is the subject of widespread diversity in terms of the institutions that organise and employ procedures and staff in the governance of research. It is widely acknowledged that the composition, structure, function and accountability of research ethics committees vary widely (Postnote, 2005). This variance applies even at more specific fields of research, as in exercise, health and sports sciences, with different approval requirements across institutions and countries. This means that researchers are faced with diverse requirements of stringency and accountability.

Research in the USA is highly regulated by the federal government, through the Code of Federal Regulations (DHHS, 2005). These regulations provide for consistency of operation. This is not necessarily the case outside the USA (although Australia and Canada have similar systems), and in the UK and most of Europe social science research, for example, is currently subject to professional self-regulation or to regulation by independent institutions such as universities. An exception to this in the UK is where National Health Service (NHS) staff or patients are involved in research, where NHS property is used as a site of data collection, where NHS records are used to identify research subjects or participants or where medical intervention forms part of a suggested protocol. In these scenarios, formal ethics approval must be obtained in order to comply with the Research Governance Framework. While there is an element of overlap here, then, there is still a clear difference between the governance structures for health research and most exercise and sports science research in the UK at least.

In the UK the Department of Health issued guidance on research ethics committees in 1975, but NHS Local Research Ethics Committees (LRECs) were not established until 1991. This was followed in 1997 by the creation of Multicentre Research Ethics Committees (MRECs) to deal with the problem of studies that took place in several sites or geographical locations. The Department of Health created a Central Office for Research Ethics Committees (COREC) in 2000 and this body subsequently became part of the National Patient Safety Agency. The European Clinical Trials Directive became part of UK law in 2004 and this led to further changes in the NHS REC system, with the introduction of Type 1, Type 2 and Type 3 RECs. Briefly, Type 1 RECs deal with the first trials of new drugs in healthy volunteers, Type 2 committees review NHS research taking place in a single geographical region (known as a single domain) and Type 3 RECs look at studies that take place in more than one region or domain. Even as we write there is a further consultation taking place on more changes to the system and this information is likely to be out of date even before our book is in print, so anyone contemplating research involving the NHS in any capacity should seek advice from the COREC website (http://www.corec.org.uk/). Within universities, where most exercise and sports science research takes place, ethics approval for projects is still somewhat uncoordinated. Most UK universities, however, now have in place some type of ethics approval requirement, at least partly because of the requirements of the Department of Health (DoH) Research Governance Framework

So, the situation in the UK and Europe is changing, following the lead of the USA, Australia and Canada. For example, RECs operate within an increasingly elaborate regulatory structure at the European and UK level. The introduction into UK law of the European Clinical Trials Directive has led to the production of new regulations and guidelines and these are likely to go through further amendment in the foreseeable future. However, at present the activities of RECs in the UK are controlled by the *Governance Arrangements for Research Ethics Committees* (GAFREC; Department of Health, 2001) and the newly issued Standard Operating Procedures (SOPs) for RECs. Both the European Union (EU) Directive and GAFREC set out the roles and responsibilities of RECs in some detail. In brief they are to:

- enable relevant research of good quality;

- provide independent advice to participants, researchers, funders, sponsors, employers, care organisations and professionals on the extent to which proposals for research studies comply with recognised ethical standards;
- protect the dignity, rights, safety and well-being of all actual or potential research participants.

They act:

> primarily in the interest of potential research participants and concerned communities, but they should also take into account the interests, needs and safety of researchers who are trying to undertake research of good quality. However, the goals of research and researchers, while important, should always be secondary to the dignity, rights, safety, and well-being of the research participants.
>
> (Department of Health, 2001: 1)

While GAFREC and GCP (good clinical practice) provide the framework for ethical review, with respect to the detail of that review they express only the requirement that studies must be assessed as complying with 'recognised ethical standards'. They make little or no specific attempt to specify what these standards are. The usual starting point for anyone wishing to explore this would be the various national and international guidelines and codes, most notably the Nuremberg Code, the Declaration of Helsinki, and the guidelines issued by the Council of International Organizations for Medical Science (CIOMS).

There is little doubt that the driver for research ethics has emanated from the spheres of medicine, irrespective of the disputes as to the universality of application of the norms and guidelines that emerge in that sphere. Therefore, we start with critical consideration of the generation of research governance structures and processes that define the field of medical research governance.

Medical research ethics

As noted above, the Nuremberg Code was produced in 1949, in the aftermath of the Second World War and the trials of the Nazi doctors.[2] It deals particularly with medical experimentation (almost all the clauses start with a reference to 'The experiment') and includes statements such as:

- The experiment should be such as to yield fruitful results for the good of society, unprocurable by other methods or means of study, and not random and unnecessary in nature.
- The experiment should be so designed and based on the results of animal experimentation and a knowledge of the natural history of the

disease or other problem under study, that the anticipated results will justify the performance of the experiment.

The Declaration of Helsinki, in its 2004 version, begins with the following statement:

> The World Medical Association has developed the Declaration of Helsinki as a statement of ethical principles to provide guidance to physicians and other participants in medical research involving human subjects. Medical research involving human subjects includes research on identifiable human material or identifiable data.

It also states in various later paragraphs (not in precise order):

> The primary purpose of medical research involving human subjects is to improve prophylactic, diagnostic and therapeutic procedures and the understanding of the aetiology and pathogenesis of disease. Even the best proven prophylactic, diagnostic, and therapeutic methods must continuously be challenged through research for their effectiveness, efficiency, accessibility and quality.
>
> Medical research involving human subjects must conform to generally accepted scientific principles, be based on a thorough knowledge of the scientific literature, other relevant sources of information, and on adequate laboratory and, where appropriate, animal experimentation.
>
> Every medical research project involving human subjects should be preceded by careful assessment of predictable risks and burdens in comparison with foreseeable benefits to the subject or to others. This does not preclude the participation of healthy volunteers in medical research. The design of all studies should be publicly available.
>
> Medical research involving human subjects should only be conducted if the importance of the objective outweighs the inherent risks and burdens to the subject. This is especially important when the human subjects are healthy volunteers.
>
> Medical research is only justified if there is a reasonable likelihood that the populations in which the research is carried out stand to benefit from the results of the research.

As with the Nuremberg Code, the Declaration of Helsinki concentrates on medical research.

Finally, the CIOMS guidelines say:

> Researchers and sponsors must ensure that proposed studies involving human subjects conform to generally accepted scientific principles, are based on adequate knowledge of the pertinent scientific literature, and accord with the state of the art of research methodology and practice.

These considerations should be adequately reflected in the research protocol submitted for approval to scientific and ethical review committees and funding agencies

Ethical review. Scientific review and ethical review cannot be clearly separated: scientifically unsound research involving humans as subjects is *ipso facto* unethical in that it may expose them to risk or inconvenience to no purpose; even if there is no risk of injury, wasting of participants' time in unproductive activities represents loss of a valuable resource. Normally, therefore, ethical review committees consider both the scientific and the ethical aspects of proposed research. They must ensure that a proper scientific review is carried out.

For all biomedical research involving humans, the researcher must ensure that studies present participants with a favourable balance of potential benefits and risks. This accords, very loosely, with utilitarian thinking outlined above. Interventions or procedures that hold out the prospect of direct diagnostic, therapeutic or preventive benefit for the individual participant must he justified by the expectation that they will be at least as advantageous to the individual, in the light of foreseeable risks and benefits, as any available alternative. Risks of such 'beneficial' interventions or procedures must be justified in relation to expected benefits to the individual participant.

The obvious limitation with all three documents, for our purposes, is that without exception they deal entirely with biomedical research. This informs every consideration of scientific method, and of assessment of risk and benefit. Methods must be rigorous and scientific, following the empiricist or positivist tradition that requires the elimination of anything that is not objectively recordable. A further problem is that, although ethics committees are charged with the appraisal of the benefit, value or worth of research, compared to its risks or costs, there is remarkably little in the literature by way of any frameworks to help with this appraisal. Casarett *et al.* (2002) have attempted to develop a 'taxonomy of value in clinical research', but this again is entirely focused on bioscience. They observe that 'patients are exposed to risks in order to create valuable knowledge' and that 'a central goal of research is to produce knowledge that is "important", "fruitful" or that will have "value" '. Writing from within an American context, Casarett *et al.* argue that 'generalizability is the cornerstone of the Common Rule definition of research' and that this is crucial to the study's validity. They develop their account of value in research as defined by 'a study's potential to improve health and well-being', a view that they point out is codified in the Nuremberg Code and the Declaration of Helsinki. They further categorise this definition of value along two dimensions: immediate vs. future health value, and the population that receives this value. These identified problems of course have some bearing on the ethical conduct, and on the governance, of most exercise and sports sciences and much health research (including qualitative research in both of these areas, see Chapter 7).

So, there is wide diversity in policy and practice, between and within countries, disciplines, institutions, funders and professional bodies. Nevertheless, and despite variations in practice, it is perhaps the most commonly shared of all research ethics norms that all researchers using subjects should obtain approval for the project before data collection can commence. As mentioned before, this process varies, and it is incumbent on researchers to familiarise themselves with the local, regional and national requirements that apply to their work. When in doubt, researchers should contact their research office or their line manager. They should not proceed with data collection until they have full, unconditional ethical approval to start the work. IRBs in the USA are required to review and approve, require modifications to, or withhold approval of research involving human subjects (DHHS, 2005).

It is generally accepted that such committees are of crucial importance in regulating research and preventing abuses, since investigators should not be the sole judges of whether their research conforms with generally acknowledged ethical codes and practices. No investigator can be totally objective in the sense of being free from personal belief and conceptual bias, and the distancing and isolation of an IRB or REC, coupled with a wide range of membership, serve to improve the objectivity of ethical decision-making (Brodie and Stopani, 1990). The apparent ideal of such a board or committee might be thought to be that as captured in the delicious phrase of Nagel (1989) as the view of the world from nowhere particular in it. It gestures towards the clash of absolutist conceptions of truth and the context-dependence of meaning and understanding. Of course no such logical or sociological distance is possible in research, let alone research ethics. Yet in keeping with the objectivist *sentiment*, while necessarily falling short of transcendental objectivity, we can easily recognise the benefits of impartiality implied by external scrutiny. And there is little to argue about in that. Accepting the all-too-human judgements of RECs or IRBs, it is worth examining the practices and procedures of ethics committees to see how their aim of critical, fair and impartial review is effected.

Composition of IRBs

It has been advocated that a wide variety of expertise and skills be represented on an IRB, which can include statisticians, administrators, lawyers, ethicists and lay members (Brodie and Stopani, 1990). USA Federal Regulations (DHHS, 2005) hold that IRBs should have at least five members, from varying backgrounds, so that issues such as race, culture and gender can be sensitively considered. Where specific competencies are required, people with the requisite knowledge should be included in committee deliberations. Non-discriminatory efforts should be made to include a gender mix, at least one member should have no affiliation with the institution, and no IRB may consist entirely of members of one profession. One member must be primarily concerned with science, and at least one member's primary concerns must be in non-scientific areas.

It has been argued that an ethics committee should include in its membership someone trained in philosophical ethics. However, a recent USA-based study found that less than a third of IRBs surveyed had a formally trained bioethicist or philosopher in their membership (Hoffman *et al.*, 2000).

If we were to accept the preceding recommendations (and many of our institutions do), then we may end up with committees of unmanageable size, meeting for extraordinarily long sessions, endlessly debating a variety of opinions that are not always relevant to the advancement of knowledge.[3] We contend that it is considered desirable to establish smaller IRBs or RECs that are staffed by well-trained individuals, rather than by a large number of merely well-intentioned ones. By 'well trained', we mean something like the following. The composition of the committee should include person(s) formally trained in moral philosophy or applied ethics. We acknowledge that, as with other aspects of ethics review, consistency of training, and implementation, will be difficult if not impossible to achieve. Nevertheless, we contend that a knowledge of moral philosophy improves the ethical decision-making process in terms of clarity, scope and consistency of evaluation. Equally, there should be representation by those familiar with the methods that the IRB or REC review, so that there is familiarity with the pitfalls that the research methods may give rise to. It may be necessary also to have some representation from research contexts – such as mental health professionals, or professionals with paediatric expertise. Often consideration must be made at a local level in relation to whether such persons should be core staff or simply co-opted members for specific proposals. If a university has no medical school and does not engage in clinical research, why include a general practitioner as a core member? If it has no engineering department, why include an engineer?

The committee should preferably be of manageable size (USA Federal Regulations require at least five members with varying backgrounds), should have the power to co-opt additional members with specific expertise for particular meetings,[4] and should be provided with adequate administrative support. In an ideal world, membership of IRBs or RECs should be taken into account by institutions when calculating workloads and remission for time spent in preparatory reading. Duration of membership should be a renewable period of something like 3–5 years. Equally, it is desirable for there to be rolling terms of office for members (say by odd and even years) so that there are not wholesale changes in the membership of the board or committee. This seemingly lengthy period is necessary for members to absorb the ethos and to develop skills and sensitivities necessary for ethical review. Where possible, each IRB/REC should have at least one senior, experienced researcher as a member. Such an individual's knowledge of regulations, processes and decision-making will not only expedite proceedings, but also serve as an educative process for less experienced members. A final possibility for membership is that of an insurance officer of the institution, for there will be legal and financial implications of formal approval, rejection and research misconduct. The success of the ethics review process depends on the standards and capability of the decision-makers, and IRBs/RECs should be trusted by society generally and by the research communities specifically.

Duties, functions and scope of IRBs/RECs

Very considerable tensions arise when considering the extent to which evaluating the technical (e.g. methodological) merit of a study is within the purview of IRBs/RECs. In this sense the role of IRBs/RECs has changed. Arising from what might be called the medical ethics paradigm, they were primarily concerned with issues surrounding the preservation of subjects' autonomy, such as the informed consent process and confidentiality. The role of research project approval committees has expanded, however, to include issues not specifically related to participant autonomy, to the extent that a broad range of design issues is now included in many discussions (Rosnow *et al.*, 1993). This too, in the UK at least, has followed the scope that RECs have had in relation to health and medical research that has gone through NHS regulatory frameworks. They may, for example, conduct in their peer review matters that do not directly relate to right action: a statistical review, an examination of compensation claims or subject complaints. In addition to this extended scope, their functions extend to issues such as the potential need to enforce sanctions against offenders, and perform any combination of these and other related functions. So, IRBs/RECs are paying increasing attention to the methodology of the studies and the relevance/significance of the topic, as well as the competence of the investigator/s in the proposed areas of study.

The shift from a narrow ethics evaluation to a broader methodological scrutiny is reflected by Jago and Bailey (2001), in their discussion of children in exercise, sports and medical research. They contend that an important part of submission to an IRB is an evaluation of the scientific validity of the study, including the statistical analysis. There is not widespread agreement on this issue. Indeed, to the contrary, there is widespread dispute. Qualitative researchers typically complain that research bias for positivistic design can allow the extended scope of research ethics committees to reinforce their own scientistic preconceptions. This bias might manifest itself in different ways. The committee might look inappropriately for statistically driven methods, or epidemiological orientations, or conformity to clinical standards (i.e. double-blind studies) that may be inappropriate for the research problem at hand and which might be better interrogated, for example, by snowballing techniques, or by focus groups, or by surveying particular groups of participants in a non-representative way. Of course, positivisitically inclined members may argue that this is not proper or real or hard science.

Irrespective of research bias by members, there is a deeper point with ethical significance here. If it is said that all research must aim toward some benefits, it is reasonable to expect that – at least on the face of it – the ends of the research aim at beneficial goals. This much conceded, it is perfectly reasonable to ask that the research problem can indeed be probed appropriately by the methods proposed. There is not an algorithm here. Jago and Bailey (2001) may well go too far, however, in their proposal when they state (as the first four of sixteen questions for the researchers preparing to submit their proposal to the reviewing board/committee):

1   Is the correct question being asked?
2   Can this study answer that question?
3   Will the study provide valuable knowledge?
4   Are there enough participants for statistical analysis?

The first three questions are derived, with minor alterations, from Nicholson (1986: 118), while they also cite Nicholson as the source of statistical requirements within proposals involving children. Moreover, it is necessary to bear in mind that Jago and Bailey are discussing these parameters in relation to paediatric research participants. Nevertheless, there is wider significance to them. These questions clearly aim to push the researcher (and guide the members) to an evaluation of the potential of the research proposal in terms of the widely applied ethical notion of beneficence. Nevertheless, even this portion of their list is problematic. Consider the following. What sense are we to make of question 1: how would researchers know if it was 'the' correct (note: singular) question that was being asked. Surely there are many that are relevant to any and every project. Something much more subtle needs to be teased out. A potential, though necessarily open-ended, question might be: 'to what extent is (are) the question(s) being addressed worthwhile?' This question can help to sharpen up responses to the questions of beneficence. Given that research will typically use resources (which may rely in whole or part on public funding in European universities at least), the following questions need to be asked: 'To what extent does it replicate current studies and/or aim to falsify aspects of extant research?' and 'Do the aims of the study go beyond the personal development of the researcher?' This last question is entirely appropriate if an undergraduate student research proposal is being developed. It would clearly be unfair to saddle such research with more substantial aims. Though where, perhaps, the research is part of a wider project, or there is an intention to publish, this question may require a stronger answer. Conversely, the bar is properly set higher for established researchers from postgraduate students and above.

The second question posed by Jago and Bailey is much more promising: The study will be wasteful of resources, at whatever level it is conducted, if the aims and methods are not coherent. Clearly some grasp of the internal coherence between the research problem, its specific questions and the methodological design is relevant to the question of beneficence. The third question, aimed at establishing a positive evaluation of the potential for benefit by the research, is perhaps the most problematic. Clearly all researchers will aspire to the production of 'valuable knowledge'. The problem is not so much with the goal but rather with its instantiation: precisely what is to count as valuable knowledge? To whom must it have value? For how long? With how much directness or immediacy of application? To be fair, that particular list could be developed very substantially. Nevertheless, if it is the job of research ethics committees to evaluate proposals against these kinds of open-ended criteria – and it surely is – then it is incumbent upon them to offer criteria that will guide researchers as to how the rules will be interpreted and the ways in which the board or committee will typically interpret them, with some relatively clear examples. This point is one often made against codes of conduct more generally: that these are more than punitive functions or powers and that they should be seen generally as a tool of professional development and a statement of professional standards which are likely to be the basis of trust therein (McNamee, 1988). We discuss this further below ('Regulation by codes of conduct', pp. 61–3).

Increased sensitivity to ideas of accountability, public scrutiny, and heightened awareness and concern for individual rights means that it is likely that the functions of IRBs/RECs will continue to expand. These committees, for example, are the bodies that will have to deal with sensitive issues introduced by developments in knowledge and technology in exercise and particularly in sports science with elite populations, e.g. drug use, ergogenic aids or even genetic engineering.

To avoid over-bureaucratisation and to streamline the approval process, ethics committees must clarify their remit – are they 'ethics' committees or 'research methods' committees, or both? The types of questions that they address must be clearly communicated to those who submit proposals in order to avoid unnecessary delays between submission and the commencement of projects. The extent to which the American College of Sports Medicine (ACSM), the British Association of Sports and Exercise Sciences (BASES), the European College of Sports Science (ECSS), or even their discipline-specific professional organisations such as the American Psychological Association (APA) or the British Sociological Association (BSA) publicly state their view of such matters will be a marker as to how seriously these organisations really do take the issue of research ethics more globally.

The effectiveness of research ethics review and the restrictive nature of IRBs/RECs

It has been contended that a sort of 'cost–benefit' process often dominates ethical decision-making in research, and that due consideration is seldom given to the ethical implications of the failure to conduct research that may be ethically ambiguous (Rosnow, 1990). This supports the view that, in the proper concern for the welfare of participants/subjects, the pendulum has swung so far that it sometimes may seriously prejudice the ability of the study to yield scientifically valid and reliable research (Kabat, 1975). This sort of concern may, at least in part, be due to the increase in legal and administrative constraints that severely limit the autonomy of university administration and the freedom of research workers (Price, 1978). Among such constraints are included the existence and machinations of IRBs/RECs, which have been perceived by some researchers as impeding research by introducing unnecessary delays and constraints (Azar, 2002). To these academics, research ethics governance is a luxurious indulgence or a wasteful barrier to efficient research. Particular resistance is often registered by academics engaged in contract research that often requires very tight turnaround times.

Social responsibility and sensitivity to individual rights must of course be recognised in scientific inquiry, but this very general notion is plagued with difficulties regarding decisions on specific issues (Kroll, 1993). Given the heterogeneous composition and size of IRBs/REC's (see earlier), legislated policies or guidelines are difficult to interpret and apply consistently. There appears to be great variability in the standards invoked and the recommendations put forward by IRBs/RECs (Rosnow *et al.*, 1993). Such inconsistencies might be traced back to the composition of the boards or committees, to differing levels of technical expertise, or it may stem from the nature of committee action and interaction. Often in a committee, an otherwise acceptable proposal may be picked up for one issue which is not crucial, then as it is being discussed the conversation throws up new issues for members and before long a momentum of critical discussion develops and the proposal becomes jeopardised. While inconsistent standards create the appearance, if not the possibility, of injustice, attention must be paid to important differences between the researchers themselves (their experience, their methodological approaches), the members and previous precedents. When, therefore Jago and Bailey write: 'Different local ethics and research committees viewed similar research in different ways' (2001: 534), we should not automatically infer that there is some bias or unfairness occurring. True, what may be reflected is a perception of inconsistent judgements on the part of IRBs/RECs,[5] but the issue goes deeper than that, with a growing perception among researchers that IRBs are increasingly acting as a 'police force' (Rosnow *et al.*, 1993). This point of view is strongly propounded by Mosher (1988: 379), who states that: 'The institutionalisation of IRBs or HSCs creates a growing bureaucracy that chills science by reducing creative nonconformity.' Whether the research community is better disposed to research governance at this time is a moot point. There are some grounds for believing (hoping?) that in the UK at least there has been a softening of attitudes and that researchers are coming to realise that ethical approval is now an obligatory part of the research process for researchers from many spheres of academia – not just medicine.

If ethics committees are to play a positive role in advancing science and

scholarship more generally, caution should not be abandoned. The likelihood of dangers and harms, however, should also not be exaggerated. This is
particularly the case for research that generally poses little physical or mental
risk, which might include much of the research performed in sports science.
For example, Jago and Bailey (2001) seem to imply that, before making a
submission to an IRB/EC, an investigator should be satisfied that the project
involves no more than negligible risk. But it is not quite clear what 'negligible
risk' entails, or indeed whether such a high threshold should be used generally or only in relation to children and other vulnerable populations (see
Chapter 7). Should we, for example, not expose participants or subjects to
procedures that are more risky than those they face travelling to the laboratory, such as crossing the road? This is tendentious, and implementation
of such guidelines unilaterally would have the consequence that very little
research would get done. A more useful instruction to both researchers and
IRBs/RECs would seem to be to perform at least some proto-utilitarian
analysis. Committees should of course take great pains to quantify and then
minimise risk, but to insist on no more than negligible risk would surely
retard the advancement of knowledge.

When a research project is delayed, either through unnecessary bureaucracy or exaggerated caution, it could be argued that the principle of human
subject protection has been misappropriated. As Mosher (1988: 379) states,
'Cover your ass is not an ethical principle.' The principle of respect for
persons should in cases such as these be applied to both participants and
researchers alike. The argument, then, is that the oppressive outside legislation represented by IRBs/RECs will cut down on both the quantity and
quality of research. Scientists claim that the spectacular growth of the 'ethics
business' has resulted in its exploitation, to the point where the application
of ethics has become unethical. Bok recognised this possibility early on in
the development of research governance when she stated:

> The bureaucracy of regulation of research can weigh as heavily as all
> other bureaucracies, and impede legitimate activity as much. Paradoxic-
> ally, it can then allow genuine abuses to slip by unnoticed in the flood of
> paperwork required and minute rules to be followed.
>
> (Bok, 1978a: 118)

The preceding sentiments are strongly supported more recently by Pettit
(1992), who feels not only that ethical review is endangering valuable research
on human beings, it is also endangering the very ethic that is needed to
govern such research. He is pessimistic about the direction that the ethical
review process is taking and feels that the reactive dynamic in operation will
lead to a serious reduction in the scope of research and to a substantial
compromise of the ethic that currently governs research practice.

With ethics committees becoming increasingly conscious of litigation,
many types of research projects are endangered, including biomedical

experiments, studies dealing with any sort of confidential information (no matter how secure the measures are), those that involve some invasion of privacy, those that include deception in the methodology, and those where subjects are unable (for a variety of reasons) to give personal consent. Pettit (1992) feels that, given this intrusion into research by IRBs, there will be increasing resentment and alienation on the part of researchers, who may come to pour scorn whatever restrictions are laid down. In this way, the restrictions insisted on by IRBs will demoralise researchers, and will lead to a restriction in the commitment of researchers to research ethics that currently prevails.

There is thus some pessimism about the effect of IRBs on research practice, and Pettit (1992: 107) feels strongly that 'there is no regulation like self-regulation'. It is tempting to agree with this, and self-regulation is of course a necessary condition for the effective functioning of research ethics, but unfortunately not a sufficient one. However, 'professionals have exhibited a pervasive inability to regulate themselves . . .' (Bok, 1978a: 118). Self-regulation does not suffice, and researchers should be held accountable, not only to their colleagues, but to all who are at risk or their representatives (Bok, 1978a).

So, we need outside scrutiny and regulation. The disadvantages of IRBs are outweighed by the benefits of careful planning, close adherence to the scientific ethic, and protection for subjects and researchers. The positive benefits should however be supplemented by realisation on the part of committees that part of their remit is the advancement of research.

IRBs should protect research participants and encourage the pursuit of new knowledge. An over-emphasis on the former when it is not necessary will retard the latter. The remit and submission requirements of committees should be clear, and should be communicated to researchers. The principles on which they are founded are very widely acknowledged. The way that their business is conducted is not always accorded the same respect.

Regulation by codes of conduct

Self-regulation, so long the only form of governance in exercise, health and sports sciences, is not a sufficient condition for the ethical practice of research. In the impulse to formalise procedures and regulations codes of conduct – particularly through the 1990s – seemed to sprout up everywhere. It is surely the case, however, that the mere existence of a code of conduct for an association could never have fooled researchers into thinking that it provided a guarantee that members of that association conduct ethical research.

Many professional bodies have such codes. They are almost always deontological (duty-based) in nature, stressing obligations and suggesting guidelines for conduct (with such conduct not necessarily confined to research contexts). They typically attempt to regulate conduct, prescribe actions and suggest guidelines for behaviour.

It has been suggested that reliance on a professional code of ethics represents a moral discourse, as it focuses on individual agency and the personal responsibility of the researcher for the relationship with participants (Ashcroft, 2003). It is precisely this 'individual' notion though, that we feel is the primary weakness of thinking that a code provides for moral action. For while codes might provide a framework for attempting to prevent non-moral action, their very utility in terms of ease of use does not promote ethical engagement with the topic in question. Put differently, if my professional code says 'You should not XYZ', then why should I question whether XYZ is right or wrong? After all, competent and deep thinking professionals have already decided the issue for me. Not only does this result in stagnation in moral thinking among people who ought to practise it, but it also stubbornly ignores contextual factors that might be important in the heterogeneous research contexts that characterise exercise, health and sports sciences.

Consider the issue of where one is to seek professional guidance, or at least not contravene a relevant professional code. What would happen, say, if I was a member of ACSM and BASES and there appeared to be inconsistent prescriptions or proscriptions on the number of blood samples one might reasonably take from a child participant? Might I simply assert in the informed consent process that my research conformed to the standards of my relevant professional organisation (without stating which was being invoked or making the participant aware of the potential conflict?) This scenario is realistic since a problem inherent within codes of conduct is that is that they are generally made up of rules, and rules (even ethically significant ones) can and do conflict. In the scenario above the person with the legalistic mindset manoeuvres the rules to his satisfaction, and thereby denies legitimacy to his actions.

It has been thought by code writers, and certain philosophers, that one can merely appeal to higher rules. Yet structuring rules hierarchically does not really work because one needs to be aware of situational factors as we saw in Chapter 2. Moreover, one has to recognise that codes are often a 'moral pastiche' (McNamee, 1998) of ideas that are important in themselves, but which draw from different ethical traditions and are thus – at times – incommensurable. Moreover, we must recognise that the forms of guidance or instruction by rules is extremely heterogeneous (Pincoffs, 1986; McNamee, 1998).

Finally, codes very rarely give guidance on how to resolve problems when their guidelines are in seeming opposition or when it is unclear how they should be applied. And, as Wittgenstein (1953) famously noted, there are no rules that apply themselves. Thus there are also, and unavoidably, differences in interpretation between individuals, and when this is allied to contextual or practical difficulties in research situations, it becomes apparent that codes, *per se*, are not sufficient to ensure the ethical conduct of research.

One final point worth making in relation to professional membership and codes of research conduct arises in the conflict between exercise and sports sciences of a positivistic bent, which draws upon the medical research tradition that elevates the notion of informed consent to an inviolable principle (which we discuss in Chapter 8). Most social science research disciplines (including sociology of exercise, health and sport) do not place academics under an obligation to join a professional body. Nor, in most instances, is there any means of disciplining individuals who do not adhere to a code in a particular discipline. Fleming noted how, as a sociologist, he had engaged in deceptive sociological research as a participant observer – a method not entirely uncommon in sociological research. Yet in doing so he fell foul of a rule of BASES of which he was also a member, in the Open Section.[6] The rule in question was a particularly severe one, which obliged members who knew of such infraction to blow the whistle on colleagues. It merited the sanction of expulsion from the association. Having blown the whistle on himself to the relevant persons he encountered nothing but apathy. What, one might reasonably ask, is the point of so severe a sanction when it is ignored by the professional association, and when it can in principle expel members for research conducted within professional norms?

Benefits of ethics scrutiny

While there are issues with the way in which the ethics scrutiny process operates, including perceptions that it creates more work for researchers and that it involves unnecessary bureaucratic delays, ethics review clearly has positive benefits for subjects, researchers and for society. Self-regulation is not sufficient to prevent research abuses, and ethics scrutiny serves the crucially important function of minimising risk and harm. In addition to protecting subjects, a system of properly conducted ethics scrutiny and approval also gives protection to researchers if something goes wrong in a study. The approval process has an educative benefit in that it forces researchers, at least to some extent, to engage with and foresee ethical problems that might be encountered in their studies. Similarly, the review process might identify and raise legitimate issues that might otherwise have been overlooked. It can also give researchers confidence that, having been approved, their studies are worthwhile and properly constructed. A properly conducted approvals process can, through avoiding scandals, engender public confidence in science as a whole, with such confidence ultimately translating to continued public participation (not least in terms of subject volunteers). Nevertheless, the concerns that researchers have about the ethics review process are real and need to be addressed.

Challenges and responses

The nature of research is changing, as is the ethics system that regulates it. For example, large multi-centre experiments and collaborative research projects are now more common. This has imposed additional stresses on the review system. In the UK, regional multi-centre research committees were established in 1997 for the NHS system of research governance. Unfortunately, there is some evidence to suggest that this has neither alleviated administrative delays nor reduced financial costs (Flynn *et al.*, 2000; Lux *et al.*, 2000; Tully *et al.*, 2000).

In the USA, there has been an increase in federal regulatory actions taken against IRBs. Federal review panels have also called for major modifications to the regulations governing IRBs. A recent editorial in *The Lancet* (2001) contends that the increased regulatory efforts have been misdirected, and that IRBs have become preoccupied with procedural matters.[7] 'If the modified system remains bureaucratic, the problems will remain' (*The Lancet*, 2001). When concerns such as these are allied to those of inconsistent judgements, it becomes clear that we need to re-evaluate the role and functions of IRBs.

Rosnow *et al.* (1993) feel that not only should IRB decisions be more consistent, but also that the power of these committees should be limited. IRBs should take into consideration not only the costs of doing research, but also the potential costs of not doing it. This would go some way to ensuring that there will be no cessation of studies that need to be done to answer important scientific and societal questions. This supports the earlier view of Stetten (1975), who contends that the fact that a problem may be difficult, or that its solution may prove politically embarrassing or unpopular, is insufficient ground for invoking constraint. Further, he holds that a science that shies away from a line of inquiry merely because the result may be difficult to manage is in a sorry state.[8]

Different strategies are needed in the face of moral problems posed by scientific investigations involving humans. First, we need agreement on what forms of research are risk-free, and then unnecessary bureaucratic impediments must be removed from such research. This approach is in line with the plea by Rosnow *et al.* (1993) for consistency in decision-making, and is also strongly supported by Pettit (1992), who feels that it is important that ethics committees concern themselves only with research projects that raise genuine difficulties. Second, we need agreement on what forms of research involve clear-cut abuse or recklessness, and we need to set clear standards, so that scientists can know beforehand when experimentation is too intrusive or too dangerous to be undertaken.

This of course leaves us with a third set of research proposals – those complex problems where disagreement persists. The challenge of the first two strategies, as Bok puts it, is to 'press the limits of the clearly intolerable and the clearly innocuous so as to make this middle group as small as possible, in order to avoid as much unnecessary dispute as we can' (1978a: 126).

Making ethical decisions

Ethics committees adopting a casuistic approach will incorporate a mix-
ture of utilitarian (consequence-based) and deontological (rights-based)
approaches in their deliberations. They are likely to be informed in this by
virtue-theoretical considerations and at times by others, including feministic
or overtly justice- or democratic-orientated political ideas. Included in evaluations as to the ethical merits of studies should be the following: the results
should be important (utilitarian); the risk–benefit ratio should be favourable
(utilitarian); voluntary informed consent should be obtained (deontological);
and considerations such as privacy, cultural factors, confidentiality and
deception should set limits on the conduct of research (deontological). As
presented above, the utilitarian conditions could be viewed as necessary but
not sufficient conditions for research to proceed. Likewise, the unjustified
absence of any of the deontological concerns may morally invalidate research
that satisfies the utilitarian criteria.

The practical implication of this is that, in any codification of research
ethics for exercise, health and sports sciences, priority ought to be assigned
to principles based on duty, rights and obligations. This deontologically
driven approach is consistent with Zelaznik's (1993) contention that the
use of humans in research is a privilege, and that the rights of research
participants ought to outweigh the desire of researchers to conduct research.

One of the potential problems identified earlier in the way IRBs operate
was the unequal distribution of reward and punishment for decisions. This
might be overcome by some sort of appeal procedure, whereby a researcher
can gain review of a negative decision. This would not only strengthen the
position of researchers (and, necessarily, research *per se*), but would also
combat the trend of IRBs becoming over-restrictive.

A practical problem here is that of time, with researchers often feeling
rightly aggrieved at a delay over a relatively insignificant issue, perhaps, for
example, related to design or statistics. Particularly at tertiary institutions,
where research is often 'in house', committees should give some thought
to granting a right of appearance to researchers if there are any questions
that need clarification.[9] Where such procedures are practically possible, the
researcher becomes relatively empowered and unnecessary delays may be
avoided. Of course, if a researcher elects not to be available for consultation
at the time of a specific meeting, then culpability for delays shifts away from
the committee and towards the researcher.

Conclusion

There are problems with the ways in which IRBs/RECs operate. Perhaps
the ethos of IRB/REC decision-making needs to be reshaped so that, primarily through educative efforts, an ethos of research ethics that is partially
independent of committees is nurtured. The remit and composition of IRBs

needs to be examined, and all scientists would support measures that introduce consistency and limit grey areas. The autonomy of research participants should continue to be highly valued, but the cost of not performing valuable research should also be factored into the decision-making process. Within the framework of the above, individual professions/disciplines could have ethical codes or guidelines, that, if carefully formulated and applied, would reduce the number of potential problems. Deontological and utilitarian considerations should shape the decisions of ethics committees but not to the exclusion of other considerations that we highlighted in Chapter 2. In the decision-making process, duties and rights will typically be accorded primacy, but the consequences to all concerned should not be ignored. The practices of these committees may be restrictive, and should be evaluated and perhaps reshaped, but the imperfections of the concept should not lead to the process being discarded.

4 Respectful research

Why 'tick-box consent' is not good enough

Against the grain of research ethics development generally, and biomedical research ethics specifically, Onora O'Neill has recently written:

> Some commonly cited reasons for thinking that informed consent is of great importance are quite unconvincing: informed consent has been supported by poor arguments and lumbered with exaggerated claims.
>
> (O'Neill, 2003: 1)

When a philosopher with the reputation enjoyed by O'Neill begins a research article with such a robust claim, the weight of justification falls on authors such as ourselves to specify more clearly the nature and importance of the concept and indeed its scope. We might think of events such as those in Dachau or indeed in Tuskegee as limit cases. These are surely about as bad as research ethics abuses get, or so we might think. But what relevance have they to everyday mundane research it could be asked? Of course, it will be said, individuals should have the freedom of choice to decide on their participation in research. That is the whole point of having informed consent. While flagrant abuses of informed consent may not be especially prevalent, it is nonetheless true that the principle and its underlying concept 'autonomy' can rather easily be offended by a failure to consider properly the concepts at hand and how they are operationalised in research. The aims of this chapter are, first, to discuss the concept of autonomy that is presupposed in informed consent and, second, to critically illustrate how it is observed and/or undermined in exercise, health and sports research. We shall then discuss the nature and ethical status of deception. This will allow us to consider what is often assumed in physiological research, for example, that informed consent is an inviolable principle and the bedrock of all research ethics whether natural or social scientific.

What is autonomy and why is it important?

There are very few nations in the Western world that do not subscribe to the value of autonomy. To put it that way might make the reader think that its scope is universal. That would be a mistake. There are cultures in the modern world that do not believe it to be the most important principle upon which to order lives and societies. We shall return to this idea specifically in our remarks on transcultural research in Chapter 10. For the moment, we must recognise the importance of the fact that the concept of autonomy is enshrined in Western ethics and indeed in international legal frameworks such as the UN Declaration of Human Rights. But what is this thing called 'autonomy'?

As with any concept there is a variety of definitions. Perhaps we should say there is a variety of conceptions because the differences they reveal are not merely a matter of trifling with language but rather with whole worldviews. This is not the place to offer an extended analysis of those differences but we can say that it is helpful to begin with some etymological remarks. The word autonomy is derived from ancient Greece where it was taken to refer to self-governance (i.e. *autos* = self; *nomos* = rule). Its original meaning was located in political contexts where it referred to the independence of *polis*: small city states such as Athens, Sparta or Corinth. Only later was its usage extended to self-governance by individuals, as we take for granted today. Its use then, over centuries and in diverse cultures, has taken on a variety of meanings as from independence of mind and being responsible for one's own actions, choices and values to individual rights to privacy and beyond.

For our purposes it is only necessary to offer a thin account of autonomy, which will help us to understand and interpret the vagaries of informed consent. John Stuart Mill set forward a philosophical *locus classicus* in his discussion of 'liberty'. He wrote:

> If a person possesses any tolerable amount of common sense and experience, his own mode of laying out his existence is the best, not because it is the best in itself, but because it is his own mode.
>
> (Mill, 1962: 197)

Here he followed that other great British utilitarian Jeremy Bentham in defining freedom as the absence of coercion. The concept of autonomy is a cornerstone of liberal politics and its nature is tied closely to that of negative liberty (Berlin, 1968). Freedom, in the liberal worldview, is essentially a freedom *from* constraints or interventions by other persons or institutions. More broadly, though, Skorupski (1991) notes that if we consider what it is that we value, autonomy is an important human end as it is:

> the freedom to determine and follow our own projects, free from the interference of others – to the extent that those projects do not affect others in ways to which they could properly object.
>
> (Skorupski, 1991: 355)

Few would disagree with the idea that autonomy has both negative and positive aspects in conceptual terms. So let us agree, regardless of our political commitments, that to act autonomously is to act in the absence of external pressures or constraints. In its positive aspect, autonomous persons must be able in some adequate sense to have come to their actions and choices as a result of understanding what lay before them. We shall note then, in summation, that autonomy (in whatever theory) should observe conditions of (1) freedom from controlling influences; and (2) agency, or the capacity for intentional action. This of course leaves open an enormous array of philosophical interpretations of these two components that we cannot address here.[1]

Commonly, the importance of the concept of autonomy is brought under the rubric of 'respect'. Many people choose to observe this rather open-ended principle as a foundation for their own ethics. This has clear relations to the deontological theories of ethics and was central to Kant's moral philosophy as discussed in Chapter 2. In keeping with its negative and positive aspect, we might think that conforming to the demands of autonomy might issue in specific course of action for researchers. These might include: (1) telling the truth about the research; (2) respecting the privacy of those who do not wish to participate in the research; (3) preserving anonymity and ensuring confidentiality; (4) obtaining consent; and (5) assisting others to make informed decisions if invited.[2]

As with all important moral notions, we need to understand autonomy in relation to its close conceptual cousins. Respecting autonomy is a critical general stance in research ethics as it is in life, leaving people to make their own decisions about the shape of their lives. But it is not the inviolable principle that some think it is. This is partly because of the nature of autonomy and partly of our human being. We are all of us, if MacIntyre (1999: 1–10) is to be believed, 'dependent rational animals'. And as Baier (1993) has observed, it is easy to fall into the trap of taking mature adults as the basis of ethical discussion. Of course it is the case that autonomy is not an on–off concept. It exists in degrees. Yet even if one disagrees with MacIntyre, no-one can seriously dispute the idea that the very old, the young and those with learning disadvantages *may* not be capable of fully autonomous choice. And this has important implications for work with and on vulnerable populations. This is discussed in detail in Chapter 8 on vulnerable participants in research. For our part, we must consider then what is and ought to be the case when confronted with the possibility of non-autonomous choice. To do this we must consider the concept of 'paternalism'.

Paternalism

The term 'paternalism' has Latin roots. In his discussion of liberty and paternalism, John Stuart Mill writes:

the sole end for which mankind are warranted, individually or collectively, in interfering with the liberty of action of any of their number, is self-protection. That the only purpose for which power can be rightfully exercised over any member of a civilised community, against his will, is to prevent harm to others. His own good, either physical or moral, is not a sufficient warrant.

(Mill, 1962: 135)

When Mill (1962) proposed categorical bans on certain patterns of behaviour that he believed were unacceptable, he influenced early definitions of paternalism to have a narrow meaning, concentrating on coercion as a mode of protecting the coerced from harm (Dworkin, 1983; Feinberg, 1983). As similarities were recognised between the intentions behind this and other ways of promoting people's interests without their consent, the concept of paternalism expanded and, in the process, came to include some clearly beneficial actions. More recently Dworkin has characterised paternalism as 'the interference with a person's liberty of action justified by reasons referring exclusively to the welfare, good, happiness, needs, interests of values of the person being coerced' (1971: 108). One of the effects of this reconceptualisation has been a recognition by some that a categorical ban on paternalistic intervention is unnecessary and inappropriate (Kultgen, 1991). The concept of paternalism has developed to include any individual or group with the power to act on others. The fundamental goal of paternalism expanded from the protection of the person from self-harm to protection from any kind of harm and promotion of any kind of good for them (Kultgen, 1991).

In this vein, Bayles (1988: 116) states: 'A person's conduct is paternalistic to the extent his or her reasons are to do something to or on behalf of another person for that person's well being.' Bayles misses the importance of the fact that paternalism proceeds without the consent of the person on whose behalf the action is taken. Like the literature on autonomy, the nature of paternalism is similarly voluminous and it is not appropriate to attempt to survey it here (see Sartorius, 1983; Kleinig, 1984).

In relation to research contexts specifically we can say that a paternalistic act exists where the researcher uses or occupies the participant or subject without their informed consent where that act will contribute to the welfare of the researched. It should be noted further that this act could be one of omission or commission; it could include an attempt to prevent a person from doing something or to conceal information from them, just as it could be intended to promote a certain good. These categories have variously been labelled 'positive' and 'negative' (Kleinig, 1984) and 'promotive' and 'preservative' (Kultgen, 1995). Whether the researcher is justified in so acting in various contexts is another matter.

An important clarification was made by Feinberg (1983), writing in the philosophy of law when he distinguished between *soft* and *hard* paternalism.

The distinction is now a commonplace in philosophical literatures. Soft paternalism refers to justifiable interventions on behalf of a person who is not fully competent in some relevant sense. Hard paternalism refers to interventions on behalf of a person who is competent yet whose desires are justifiably overridden by another. Cases of strong paternalism are not common with mature human beings in Western liberal democracies. There are clear cases, usually referred to as 'legal paternalism', such as the wearing of seatbelts and crash helmets and the non-use of certain drugs. In medicine and the law, professionals are thought to be justified in their paternalism when this is the best or only method of assisting the client to achieve their ends. Such strong paternalism is unlikely ever to be attempted or justified by researchers. We can summarise this by saying that 'strong' paternalism overrides an autonomous person's wishes, choices or actions, while 'weak' paternalism does the same for non-autonomous persons (e.g. those with a diminished capacity for understanding the consequences of actions, or children under a certain age) (Veatch, 1989).

When, if ever, can researchers make decisions on behalf of other people? For example, are there any situations in which the researcher can proceed with a project when the subjects have not provided informed consent? Can they conduct research on a group of people, without their consent, if they feel that they know better than the participants that the research will be beneficent and will prove valuable to them and others?

A positive answer to the latter question would involve adopting a strong paternalistic position. This might particularly be the case in research if we attempted to rank consequentialist principles over non-consequentialist ones (e.g. welfare over duties, obligations or rights). Paternalistic actions might be justified, for example, where a refusal to acquiesce in a subject's or participant's wishes, choices and actions for that person's own benefit – were to their benefit (Veatch, 1989). For example, in therapeutic research, it might hypothetically be argued that a particular exercise regime will benefit Down syndrome sufferers, even if they cannot fully consent to the intervention, and perhaps clearly don't like participating. All these apparent 'impositions' are examples of researchers deciding what is best for individual participants – in effect removing autonomous choice.

If we accept this distinction, then weak paternalism does not necessarily involve conflict between beneficence and autonomy. It follows, however, that strong paternalism raises the more serious moral questions and is unlikely to be justified or even supported by relevant research ethics regulatory frameworks.

What is, and what is not, 'informed consent'?

Scientific developments and technological advances have resulted in increased ability to manipulate human participants or subjects. In exercise, health and sports sciences, procedures may involve the researcher taking blood samples and biopsies, using radioactive tracers, requiring the subject to exercise to maximum effort, or performing potentially invasive psychological procedures. Past abuses in biomedical research have resulted in legal and bureaucratic controls, which have led to certain limits being imposed on researchers (Brodie and Stopani, 1990). Such controls, as we have seen in the foregoing chapters, include obtaining informed consent and submitting projects to Institutional Review Boards (IRBs) for approval. Nevertheless, even after formal recognition of the concept of informed consent in the Nuremberg Code, the Declaration of Helsinki and the Belmont Report (1979) the application of informed consent has been widely debated.

The result of this debate is that obtaining informed consent has become an almost universal research mechanism in conducting biomedical and psychological research and has received only slightly less, though still widespread, acceptance in social scientific research. One of the lead bodies in sports sciences research, The American College of Sports Medicine (ACSM), has stated that:

> Obtaining informed consent from participants before exercise testing and participation in an exercise program is an important ethical and legal consideration.
>
> (ACSM, 2006: 49)

This is in keeping with the broader position adopted by the American legislature in the wake of the Belmont inquiry in 1978. Given the requirement of informed consent, researchers need to be aware of what the concept involves. But first it is of the utmost importance to spell out what it is *not* since it is our contention that a practice masquerading as informed consent often occupies the place of the principle proper. We shall call this 'tick-box consent'. Informed consent is often taken to have been secured when a participant or subject signs a consent form and agrees to participate in the study. Not infrequently these forms represent no more than a nod in the direction of informed consent. They may be incomplete; they may fail to include a description of the duration and frequency of requirements upon them; they may fail to specify the exact aims of the study; they may be misleading because of omissions; they may be written in specialised technical jargon so as to render understanding difficult or impossible; they may form part of a series of lectures where being part of an experiment is, or appears to be, compulsory or perceived to be advantageous to students. To gain tick-box consent is therefore to deny the participant or subject the capacity to be sufficiently informed to make an autonomous choice. This is *not* informed consent in any meaningful sense where the participant or subject is *free from* (i.e. negatively free) duress or properly informed so as to be *free to* (i.e. positive freedom) make an autonomous judgement. Sadly, many of these unethical practices still abound in research in exercise, health and sports domains.

The elements of informed consent across the research spectrum

A naïve analysis of informed consent might go something like this. There are two components to the concept: 'informed' and 'consent'. We need to understand these separately and then compound them. Thus, 'informed' implies that potential subjects (or their legal representatives) obtain sufficient information about the project. This information must be presented in such a way that it is matched to the appropriate comprehension level, enabling subjects to evaluate and understand the implications of what they are about to agree to. Second, 'consent' implies free, voluntary agreement to participation, without coercion or unfair inducement. This approach, while being a good beginning is nowhere near adequate. It also begs the fallacy of composition (Morgan, 1974), the thought that one can break down complex terms into their constituents and merely add them up, as if the sum of the parts were equal to the whole.

Recent writings have adopted a more detailed approach. Many, perhaps most, writings that analyse the precise nature of informed consent in research typically list three (Sieber, 1992) or four components (see, for example, Homan, 1991; Homan, 2002; Shrader-Frechette, 1994). The former lists voluntariness, informedness and consent, while in the latter, the principle of informed consent may be operationally expressed in four elements, two of which pertain to the information received, and the other two to the voluntariness of the consenting party (Homan, 1991: 71, reproduced in Homan, 2002: 56).

Information

1   That the relevant aspects of what will occur, and what might occur, are disclosed to the subject;
2   That the subject should comprehend the information, and its implications.

Consent

1   That the subject is able to make a rational, mature, considered judgement;
2   That the subject's agreement is voluntary, free from coercion, undue influence or threat of sanction.

We contend that these aspects of the principles of informed consent would yield a considerable improvement in practice were they to be observed. But we set our sights slightly higher here in terms of explication and recommendations for practice. To that end we consider the application of the more detailed account found in biomedical ethics, adapting and adopting the seven elements set out in Beauchamp and Childress's (2001: 80–112) account.

Threshold elements (preconditions)

1   Competence (to understand and decide)
2   Voluntariness (in deciding)

Information elements

3   Disclosure (of material information)
4   Recommendation (of a plan)
5   Understanding (of 3 and 4)

Consent elements

6   Decision (in favour of a plan)
7   Authorisation (of the chosen plan)

Given the antipathy to research ethics processes of some researchers in the various domains of exercise, health and sport, the presence of this extended list requires some explanation and justification.

One of the reasons for extending the list in this way is to capture the fact that the sciences typically aim at different standards of validity and reliability according to the topic under investigation and the methodology aimed at probing it in a scientific manner. The model we have selected has been taken as an example of best practice in biomedical research and professional practice in that sphere. A legion of qualitative researchers, sociological and psychological, may well question 'Why should it be relevant in the diverse contexts and research disciplines of exercise, health and sport?'

In the first instance we note that not all of these elements will apply equally to all research designs. The very act of disregarding one of them, however, should be the product of critical reflection not simply the assumption of inappropriateness. What would be desirable is an educated rejection not merely a dismissal based upon a lack of knowledge or mere bias.

The model, following contemporary bioethics, places a very high (though not unassailable) emphasis on the value of autonomy, but respects that value in terms of *prima facie* duties. That is to say, while researchers have obligations to respect the autonomy of research participants or subjects, there exists the possibility of negotiations against other ethical norms or values, and the possibility of alternative approaches in the ways in which the researched are engaged before and during the research process. In natural sciences no or little negotiation is typical. Participants are very often treated as mere subjects once the consent form is signed. This is perfectly reasonable in normal circumstances since the control of variables and consistency of design require that the researched *conform* to the study design. This is one way in which the term 'subject' is properly applied to those individuals who consent to be measured, observed, studied, weighed and so on. Some organisations' codes of conduct, such as that of the American Psychological Association (APA), no longer make reference to the term research subject (except with reference to non-human animals; APA, 2002).[3] Others, such as the Sport and Exercise Science of New Zealand (SESNZ) Association, despite advertising that their code was drawn up in consultation with the New Zealand Psychological Association, refer to participants in their section on research, while referring to the same as subjects when discussing athlete assessments.

In the social sciences, by contrast, there is at least typically the possibility or space for negotiation between researchers and participants. This shift in terminology from subjects to participants acknowledges at the same time a shift in the power balance (Kelman, 1972). Those researched under the label 'participants', are not thought necessarily to be inert in the processes of research.[4] The researchers have a general research problem to be investigated and this is something that is typically complex and open-ended, and its probing will relate to and even alter the behaviour of the researched. This reflexivity is something that requires acknowledgement and discussion in order to respect the autonomy of the participant. Here the use of 'participant' is justified since they are properly considered partners in the research process, despite the power imbalance that usually exists between the researcher and the researched. Notwithstanding the above remarks, it is worth noting that, while it is typically the case that the researcher is an empowered figure in relation to the researched, this is not always the case. Sometimes participants know only too well that the data they have are precious to the researcher. Participants have at times been known to call the shots and curtail their engagement in the research process according to their own agenda (see Sugden, 2005).

We shall observe this distinction, according to that rationale, throughout the rest of the book. Where we refer to participants, it will be because there is a conscious identification of the contribution the researched make to the project. We still use the term 'research subject' to denote the 'objectification' of the researched as an inert and controlled component of the research.

Competence to consent

It seems fair to say that we should think of *competence* as a logically incomplete concept.[5] It is rather like the concept of fitness in that regard. One cannot properly ask the question whether X is fit, without specifying that in relation to which he or she can be evaluated as such. Is a postdoctoral assistant fit to conduct an observational experiment unsupervised? Are you fit to perform a treadmill test? So, with the idea of competence to consent, we should not expect a global response. The question does not permit it. If we wish to know whether someone is fit to give consent, we must ask whether they are competent in the relevant sense.

Culver and Gert (1982) refer to this as task-oriented competence. For research participants or subjects to give consent they must understand what they are being asked to do before they can competently give consent. One might adopt the position that anyone capable of traversing life's vicissitudes is capable of consenting to be a research subject/participant in exercise, health or sports sciences insofar as they are informable and cognitively capable. Being informable, as White (1992: 51) notes, is not the same as being informed. The former is a capability or capacity while the latter is a positive state of affairs. At the outset of any research we must ask whether the researched are informable *and* capable of comprehension of the task at hand: in short, we must determine their competence.[6] We will return to this issue below when discussing the informational elements of informed consent ('Recommendations and understanding', p. 85).

Voluntariness and informed consent

The issue of voluntariness speaks directly to the negative aspect of autonomy: freedom from external constraints. Now, while it is clear that the Nazi experiments were carried out under direct coercion backed by ultimate force, no research in our spheres will be of that kind. We must, however, be alert to the denial of voluntariness of research subjects and participants that may take more subtle forms, such as duress or undue inducements or rewards or other unacceptable inducements or pressures that may be brought to bear on the researched. It should be noted that each professional association will have made its own declaration in regard to this important issue. The British Association of Sports and Exercise Sciences (BASES), for example, states exactly such a requirement for its members (2000: 2).

One of the chief difficulties here is determining when an inducement is 'undue' or when and influence is a 'controlling one'. While it is true that not all forms of influence are controlling ones, Beauchamp and Childress (2001: 94–8) outline three such forms of improper influence: coercion, manipulation and persuasion. It would be easy peremptorily to conclude that we could dismiss coercion as irrelevant to our concerns. Yet there are borderline cases in exercise physiology, for example, where we can ask whether coercive powers are in force. Imagine that you are an elite male football player who is being assessed via a maximal anaerobic power test along with all team members prior to the start of the new season. This will involve running to exhaustion on the treadmill at significantly high speeds. The coach has demanded of the physiologist's team and the players that absolutely accurate data are necessary. To do this, the physiologist's team know that they must create the 'right' environment for the athlete to perform at maximal level in the absence of the competitive environment or any obvious external reward. When the lead physiologist of the laboratory, a former professional footballer, sees that the research subject is nearing his maximal effort he starts to ridicule him, he calls into question his heterosexuality with homophobic remarks, finally he swears at and abuses him. The researcher's team look on in disbelief never having heard their supervisor behave in such a way. They do not feel sufficiently confident to challenge his behaviour. The subject gives his all. When he exits the sprint treadmill and the machine is switched off, the lead researcher thanks the subject and assures him that the abuse he meted out was merely to obtain valid data in terms of the proper maximal, not sub-maximal, data.

While this behaviour, which is not unheard of in many exercise physiology laboratories, achieves its ends, we must question the means by which they are secured. In what sense can the researcher be said to have respected the subject? Yet the form and the process for informed consent may have appeared to be completely standard. We may ask first whether the subject knew properly what he had consented to (a point we address in detail below) but for our purposes here we must ask whether the actions of the researcher – sanctioned by the professional's paymaster – are coercive.

If we develop the scenario a little we can see how it might go. Imagine that the next day's tests involve attempts to evaluate the football player's anaerobic endurance. This will involve several repetitions of more sustained periods of maximal effort up to 45 seconds. The treadmill is placed on an incline. The subject is wary that if he gives it his absolute all he may injure himself on the treadmill or, worse, shoot off the back if he fails to use the handrail and jump from the treadmill travelling at 25 mph. At repetition four of the six the subject vomits upon completion – a not uncommon outcome from maximal anaerobic endurance training. He states a desire not to complete the test. The researcher remonstrates with him. The subject holds his ground but is wavering. The researcher reminds the subject that the consent form made clear the nature and intensity of the test. He reminds him of the need for the researcher to complete all of the tests satisfactorily for his employer. He compares him unfavourably to other team players who have completed the test. Finally, the subject agrees. It is clear that such a scenario is not easy to describe as 'coercive'. It is more complex than cases where the subject is completely powerless. Yet it raises serious questions regarding what is acceptable in terms of motivating subjects to perform to achieve data of the greatest veracity. And it is clear that it falls far short of showing the respect that a participant or subject is typically owed. How would it square with the idea that research subjects are free to withdraw from research projects at any stage (see, among many examples of this requirement, BASES, 2000: 4)?

What we have aimed to do here is merely to plant a thought. This may well be common practice in physiological tests to identify maximal outputs. Its frequency should not give us occasion to gloss over it as 'business as usual'. Indeed, to do so will in a real sense give the lie to the moral calluses that may be part of the professional initiation of the research apprentices, whether at undergraduate or postgraduate level. It has been suggested that precisely a certain kind of environment may have been created when physiologists first attempted to carry out painful muscle biopsies using the research team (students/colleagues) on multiple occasions, as they were effectively a captive audience. Let us assume that at least tick-box consent has been gained from colleagues of the principal researcher. Can we also assume that no pressure was felt – even if it was not directly brought to bear by the research leader – by junior members of the research team to engage other research students or other colleagues?

One of the most sensible responses to issues such as these in relation to voluntariness and undue pressure has been the development of what are referred to as 'cooling-off periods'. In order to avoid the possibility of duress in situations, particularly where the relation between researcher and participant/subject is ambiguous or multi-layered (such as with students or clients), it is wise to determine a period of time when the participant or subject can reflect on their consent. During this time they can discuss with other participants/subjects or other confidants about the wisdom of participation, all things considered. It might be thought that where the participant/subject is in a relatively powerless position in relation to the researcher, or where payments are to be made, the cooling-off period is especially applicable. These cases are at the beginning of a continuum in which we can relate the researcher to the researched in terms of power-related considerations. The far end of this continuum will be occupied by participants and subjects who may be thought of as captive populations.

Voluntariness and captive populations

One of the most frequently discussed issues in this regard has been described as the 'volunteer effect' (Rosenthal and Rosnow, 1962). We shall discuss this below in relation to the ethics of using captive populations. In what follows, we focus on issues of voluntariness with respect to captive populations. We shall not treat them separately. Clearly that would be a separate task too far removed from present purposes. Carefully distinguishing among concepts such as 'duress', 'manipulation' and varieties of 'persuasion' would be a fit object for philosophical analysis but we do not attempt that task here. We content ourselves with simply charting some acts which would fall into the category of inappropriate influence.

One of the most common and effective ways of using undue influence is to use subjects/participants who are enmeshed in the same institution or organisation as the researcher. For some this is a matter of convenience, while for others it may be one of necessity. If, for example, one is a part-time researcher and is released to study on the grounds that the research topic is such that it focuses on the workplace, with co-workers, in an effort to improve working life in their school, sports club or hospital, then the choice of research site is not necessarily optional. And this will be reflected in the study's design and methodology. In other cases, often referred to as convenience sampling, the researcher (as the label suggests) utilises a range of participants/subjects who are convenient as opposed to selectively drawn to illustrate a range of cohort characteristics or to achieve some measure of representativeness from which to generalise the data collected and analysed. This type of sampling has been criticised on epistemological grounds but there are ethical considerations too that may effectively undermine the voluntariness condition of informed consent. We shall explore some varieties of this type of problem below.

Patrick (1983: 637) states that 'critical to scientific success is a ready supply of experimental subjects'. The important phrase here is 'ready supply', and it is acknowledged that recruitment is easier if one has a 'captive' population from which to draw. In the early days of kinesiological, physiological and psychological research in exercise and sports science, lecturers frequently drew upon captive student cohorts to gather significantly large volumes of data. Typically, research study cohorts were drawn from students, tournament participants, team members, school children, patients and so on. Given the potentially authoritarian nature of their situation (where we can imagine students being 'controlled' by lecturers, officials, sports team captains and coaches, teachers and medical staff respectively), such subjects may perceive an element of coercion, duress or manipulation in participation. They may even experience the perception of sanction attached to non-participation. This of course makes a mockery of the notion of voluntariness in research.

For example, a coach may say: 'Which of you would like to volunteer for a research study that determines your ability to cope with high temperatures that the team will endure in next month's fixture? The study will be useful to you and the team.' This places pressure on team members, particularly in sports that emphasise the importance of collective action and responsibility (most team sports). The pressure of potential sanction can also be applied. For example, a teacher might say: 'Would you like to volunteer to perform a physical test for researcher A? Those of you who choose not to participate can come indoors and write an essay on. . . .' These are not particularly subtle examples, but they can and do occur in the world of research, necessitating informed consent (and child assent – see Chapter 7) procedures.

In cases such as those described above, the issue becomes one of *how* free the research subjects are, rather than just one of how informed they are, and researchers need to question whether or not utility should trump the right to self-determination of participants or subjects (Olivier, 1996). One way of downgrading this possibility is with the introduction of a cooling-off period and an explanation of why such a period is helpful. This will avoid the appearance of coercion, improper reward or sanction, just as much as it will genuinely give time to the participant/subject to think the matter through appropriately and, if necessary, seek guidance from trusted others.

It is probably safer to avoid the recruitment of one's students for research, all things considered. It should certainly not be done merely as a matter of convenience for the researcher. Despite more than 25 years passing since

Liemohn offered this view, the practice was alive and well in the 1990s and has not fully been disowned. If students are necessarily the subject of research we do well to heed Liemohn's (1979) warning that, when recruiting, it must be made explicit that consent is not being sought under any duress and that it must be clearly communicated that a student's subsequent decision will have no bearing whatsoever on grades.

It is necessary for researchers to consider, then, whether the autonomous choice of participants/subjects is viewed as intrinsically valuable, rather than extrinsically – merely as a means to the researchers' purposes. In many cases, it is safe to say, the value placed on autonomy goes no further than securing the tick-box version of informed consent. O'Neill (2003: 5) has aptly labelled such a process 'performing the ritual' of informed consent. At worst it is tantamount to manipulation and abuse in order to procure subjects. The clear point that Beauchamp and Childress (2001) make in relation to health-care professionals extends *mutatis mutandis* to us as researchers: we should consider ourselves under an obligation to abstain from the use of controlling influences over our participants/subjects in order to respect their rights to autonomy.

Voluntariness and gatekeepers

A very frequent way in which voluntariness can be undermined is in the use of gatekeepers (Homan, 1991: 82–7, 2002, 2005). Many research methods texts talk about the importance of gatekeepers to the research site, whether this is a health and leisure club, day-care centre, a sporting event or a gym. They are often essential in gaining access to either a place or population, and typically both when the research extends beyond the laboratory or university: the gatekeeper literally opens the way to the researcher.

It is important to note that this very general description belies greater complexity. It is worth attending to that complexity in order to understand how things may go wrong in their use because of the differing ways in which the gatekeeper is situated in relation to the researched, the site and the researcher. There are four varieties of gatekeeper (Homan, 1991). We adapt Homan's descriptions to our purposes:

1   Gatekeepers who control spatial access that gives rise to legal and other responsibilities that demand the researcher gains formal approval to do the research (e.g. gym club owners, hospital administrators, leisure centre managers). Also in this category are included gatekeepers whose power is *not* legally sanctioned but through whom it is both expected and courteous to gain access (the captain of a netball team, the elders of a community, the representatives of an interest group, the coach of a varsity team).

2   Gatekeepers may be data users or owners. Some research involves secondary data, held by third parties, who become gatekeepers through

legal means such as the Data Protection Act in the UK. The gatekeepers are then those who originally sought consent for and hold the data.

3 Gatekeepers may act in place of vulnerable populations and give consent by proxy (such as the managers of geriatric or palliative care homes, ward nurses, coaches of youth teams, school headteachers).

4 Gatekeepers may act in place of incompetent populations, or in cultures other than those to which the researcher belongs, so as to validate the researchers' authenticity; they may ameliorate gendered or racist anxieties in the participant population, or simply reduce suspicion (such as may exist in gay and homosexual groups, religious groups, or culturally specific regions and places of association).

In relation to the owners of secondary data, issues arise of whether consent passes on from the original research to the proposed research. With respect to proxy consent, we will deal with this specifically in relation to vulnerable populations in Chapter 8, where the use of gatekeepers may be an effective means of preventing informed consent. We shall refer specifically to well-known professional guidelines in this area of consent given the potential seriousness of abuses. We shall also point out some serious inconsistencies in the guidelines about therapeutic and non-therapeutic research with children (Edwards and McNamee, 2005).

It should clear that the bypassing of legitimate gatekeepers is itself problematic. In the first instance, where legal gatekeepers are avoided legal redress may be sought. Obviously this may have implications not merely for the researcher but also potentially for the supervisory team and/or the university to which they belong. Less obviously, it may result in deep offence to the group under investigation. As with the deep suspicion that attended much psychological research in the post-war period, there may arise a cynicism that affects the general public's attitude toward engaging in research. This is brought in to focus particularly in relation to deceptive research discussed in Chapter 7.

Less dramatically, though no less importantly, the failure to approach and gain consent from appropriate gatekeepers may result in a specific population or sub-culture rejecting all approaches from the academic community itself. This issue of 'outsider research' (Bridges, 2001) has been exemplified particularly in relation to issues of disability, race and gender. We shall consider two such cases. Its assertive posture is captured in the political slogan 'nothing about us without us'. The idea that the researched populations should have their voices heard and their values and viewpoints respected has reached the stage where, in some cases, activism has effectively prevented research going ahead or stopped it in mid-flow. This has most recently happened in HIV research in Cambodia and Cameroon (Mills *et al.*, 2005).

Voluntariness and payment

Around universities one commonly sees on students' notice boards invitations to students to earn relatively small amounts of money by giving up their time to be subjects for various research projects. Is there really anything wrong with this practice? There is little unanimity concerning the practice of paying research subjects, particularly when intrusive procedures are involved. Much will depend on the nature of the payment and the risks at hand. Researchers must be satisfied that payment does not constitute coercion or undue influence. Contemporary biomedical cases have brought this issue into relief.

In a recent study of subjects in a medical school in relation to pharmaceutical research, Bentley and Thacker (2004) concluded that monetary payments make subjects more willing to participate in research. On its own this may not be thought of as particularly problematic. The same study reported that the presence of payment did not alter the subjects' responses concerning the negative effects experienced in the research. This finding should not be generalised, however, and contrasts with the warnings of Mahon (1987) and Bok (1978a). Why do people object then? Under the headings we have already discussed we might see how objections could be raised both in respect of the voluntariness and the understanding elements of informed consent (Dickert and Grady, 1999). These aspects are exacerbated when we consider socio-economic status of the volunteers themselves. We can then begin to see some equity issues that might appear troublesome (Bok, 1978; Macklin, 1981; Ackerman, 1989; Dickert and Grady, 1999). As regards the voluntary and understanding aspect, perhaps we can agree on two general norms: that payment should not adversely affect the judgement of potential subjects in respect of risk assessment and statements on payment to subjects should not deflect attention away from the other information in the informed consent form.

The problem is not equally applicable across the spectrum of research disciplines in exercise, health and sport. In an electronic search of sociology journals we found no incidence of the phrase 'payment to research subjects or participants' in major journals. By contrast, in pharmaceutical research there seems to be a universal need to incentivise research participation. Here especially there have been concerns that undue pressure is placed on participants from poorer backgrounds. There are, however, borderline issues that may be worth considering for health and exercise scientists in particular.

In a recent troubling experiment a young and otherwise healthy subject died in some clinical research on an asthma drug (Ogilvie, 2001). The day after receiving the trial drug, the volunteer experienced a range of flu-like symptoms which led eventually to multi-organ failure for which no specific aetiology was found. Interestingly, Ogilvie (2001: 1335) notes that: 'The woman had been a technician at another laboratory at the centre that gave time off work for the experiments in addition to the usual modest honorarium.' In the discussion of aftercare for participants in clinical research, Harth and Thong point to an almost inevitable conflict:

> On the one hand, society may have a moral obligation to compensate and reward some of its members who assume the risk of research subjects for the benefit of society as a whole. On the other hand, the promise of aftercare may provide an inducement to volunteers which, under certain conditions, may be considered morally wrong and scientifically unsound.
>
> (Harth and Thong, 1995: 225)

Where payment is considered unavoidable in order to obtain a viable research pool, it is worth considering two further points. First, subjects must be paid in a manner that will not be manipulative. Consideration should be given to one of three models that might be utilised (Dickert and Grady, 1999):

1   market model (where the market determines the appropriate level of payment);
2   wage payment model (based on strict equality: everyone gets the same because their contribution to the research in time and effort is the same); and
3   reimbursement model (where justice as equity [i.e. social fairness] demands that volunteers only receive expenses they incur [including time away from paid employment], which may differ).

Dickert and Grady (1999: 200) argue that the latter is to be favoured for three reasons: 'First, it precludes subjects making a profit. Second, it does not use money to compensate for nonfinancial "expenses," such as effort or discomfort. Third, payment does not depend on any market, either for research participation or for unskilled labor.' While these are valuable reasons for rejecting the exploitation that can occur in the market model, and the transformation of the researcher–subject relationship into a commercial one in the wage payment model, there are still some reservations to be made about even the reimbursement model.

There are of course non-financial benefits to the research participants that might be worth exploring. We might ask what benefits the participants in research might expect from engaging in such a study; ought it to take the form of de-brief seminars, or access to new information about pharmacological products? Increasingly, social scientists have recently attempted to boost participation by 'ethical inducements', such as contributions to registered charities. This is a welcome development and one that appears to be becoming more widespread.

Second, it should be considered an obligation of the research team to put in place relevant insurance in the event of injury as a consequence of participation (Guest, 1997). Guest goes so far as to say that because, for example, the British pharmaceutical industry has no compulsions with regard to subject compensation, LRECs should seriously entertain rejecting any research proposals that do not include satisfactory assurances regarding insurance. Compensation policies may in some cases mean no more than creating cover as part of existing university-wide policies, but this should always be checked in advance of formulating detailed proposals to Research Ethics Committees (RECs) or Institutional Research Boards (IRBs).

It seems clear that inducements will not disappear from research investigations. It is not even clear that they ought so to do. Nevertheless, all good researchers (we surmise) would acknowledge that inducements should not be coercive, exploitative or even excessive. While motivations to participate in research will always be mixed, as Diener and Crandall (1978) observed long ago, it might be foolish to attempt blanket bans.[7]

Disclosure

The issue of risk disclosure is crucial to informed consent in principle. In practice, of course, much will vary with the nature and purposes of the research and the researched population. In biomedical research it is thought critical. In certain social scientific research in exercise, health and sport (we claim), it is often glossed over since the researchers themselves presuppose that no harm is likely to ensue directly from participation. Hence they commonly ignore it. This is not acceptable in the light of the account we have given of the need to recognise and respect autonomy in informed consent. To respect the fact that the participant or subject has a right to choose whether to engage with the research, their decision should be based on all relevant information. This requires a reasonably full disclosure of risks so far as the researcher can foresee them.

The relationship between the research and the researched is, as we have noted, critical. So, for example, where subjects for an exercise science experiment know that their participation would increase their risk of a heart attack by a factor of 5 or 6 (Shephard, 1995), we can reasonably assume that this might be an important factor in their choosing whether to engage or not.

Of course, once we appreciate the principle of disclosure we have still to decide on key issues: what standard of disclosure is sufficient? Beauchamp and Childress (2001) note that there is a strong legalistic dimension to this issue. This is not surprising given our comments about insurance indemnity and compensation in the previous section. It has been suggested that risk disclosure in biomedical research comes under the same type of rubric as a doctor's duty of care to her or his patients. Redress has been sought for injury to persons or property arising from the negligent failure to disclose risk by physicians. As Beauchamp and Childress note, it was in this context that the term *informed consent* was born. We adopt and adapt their general recommendations (2001: 81) below.

Researchers should typically disclose:

1   facts or descriptions that participants or subjects would consider material in the decision to offer or withhold consent regarding the research;
2   facts or descriptions that the researcher considers material;
3   the researcher's recommendation;
4   the purpose of seeking consent; and
5   he nature and limits of consent as an act of authorisation.

Most of this list will appear commonsensical to the reader, with the exception of items 3 and 4. We will address these points, having noted the need to consider two different standards[8] of disclosure in the light of this list.

Recommendations and understanding

Having said that the information disclosed must satisfy the participant's/ subject's and the researcher's appreciation of what is material, we are still left with judgements to make. We noted this in the previous section and will now make specific points in relation to understanding. The language that the disclosure is captured in is critically important.

The matter is not as easy as it appears and there is evidence of a failure of health researchers in the USA to conform to this element of informed consent (Paasche Orlow *et al.*, 2003).[9] Similarly, recent research in the UK has shown that a substantial proportion of consent documents do not cater adequately for subjects who have low reading levels. In a study examining information leaflets given to palliative care patients in Britain, only 40 per cent of the population would have had enough understanding to give informed consent. Many of these documents did not meet basic guidelines on legibility and readability (Payne *et al.*, 2000). In sport psychology, Cardinal *et al.* (1996) found that more than 85 per cent of consent forms they examined were at a reading level termed 'difficult' or 'very difficult'.

How might we do better then? How should we decide how much information is required, and at what level it should be presented, to gain informed consent proper? Moreover, how would we know whether the participants or subjects understand the process? These questions point to a difficult, equivocal area, but gathering information on the second question will help to answer the first. Understanding a document is related to its readability, and one way of testing readability is to perform a simple electronic test, for example using the readability statistics contained in Microsoft Word or some similar programme. A better method would be to conduct a comprehension check on a representative sample of your participants/subjects (see Cardinal, 2000). The outcome of your checks should then inform your decisions on the level and amount of information that you provide to ensure that subjects make a choice that is free, and that the choice is based on sufficient knowledge.

Here are some very general suggestions that may improve readability of the informed-consent document:

1   Type forms in a 12-point font.
2   Do not justify the right-hand margin.
3   Use short sentences and paragraphs.
4   Do not use technical terms (jargon).
5   Use the active rather than the passive voice.
6   Use headings and bullet points.
7   Adjust readability for intended subjects, especially those lacking higher education.
8   Check readability statistics using the option in Microsoft Word or similar text editor.
9   Pilot test the comprehension of the form.

These very general and rather simple practices may considerably assist in the comprehension of the consent form in a way that is respectful of autonomy and avoids the ritual 'tick-box consent' that we have suggested characterises too much research in exercise, health and sports sciences.

As to the issue of recommendation, it should be clear that this aspect of informed consent is driven by the possibility of alternative modes of treatment. The application of this point finds no home in almost all research in exercise, health and sports science. There is one potential exception here. Especially where sensitive data is sought, it may be advisable for the researcher to consider the modes of data collection, analysis and reporting with the researched. Here what is sought is a form of negotiation with the participant. This is discussed further in Chapter 7. What, then, of the standards of interpretation of the informational elements of informed consent?

First, there is the *reasonable person* standard. Here the researcher appeals to a hypothetical reasonable person. It must be noted that common sense hides many prejudices. Precisely what the researcher feels is the standard of a reasonable person is a moot point. Nonetheless, the standard is (somehow) widely employed. Second, there is a *subjective standard* of disclosure. The label here is misleading and unhelpful. In some philosophical circles the term would be considered oxymoronic: if it is subjective, it may be said, there can be no public standards of disclosure. What is meant by this standard is that, in contrast to a general hypothetical other (the reasonable person), information must be tailored to the individual whose consent is sought. Here the researcher ought to consider any unusual or uncommon beliefs, habits or health problems that the individual presents in virtue of their individuality and or cultural/religious membership. It should be noted that while this standard clearly represents an improvement on the former because of its specificity, it alone is insufficient. A professional judgement is unavoidable, and clearly the researcher must reconcile some combination of the two, according to the demands of the participants/subjects and the nature of the research.

Earlier we noted, with regard to recommendations with regard to disclosure, that point 3, the researcher's recommendation, and point 5, the nature and limits of consent as an act of authorisation, needed to be amplified. We turn to those issues now.

Decision and authorisation

Researchers must decide the form that the decision to withhold or give consent must take. Written consent is now considered to be the norm for all but the most minor of research procedures (see, e.g., BASES, 2000: 2). As we have tried to indicate, written consent, although necessary, is not sufficient if we are to avoid the tick-box mentality. Clearly this general peroration to view consent as a process and not a on-off event will alter according to the potential risks associated. An example may help here.

One of the authors was involved in a sprint treadmill laboratory experiment (Ramsbottom *et al.*, 1994, 1997). The lead researcher was clearly concerned about the possibilities of harm to participants (called 'subjects') who – in order to give maximal data – would run to exhaustion, which seriously involved the possibility of cramp or considerable discomfort which could cause injury while running on the treadmill at (relatively) high speeds. In order to assure himself that no harm would come to the participants, and that the participants had consented with full understanding of the process and its risks, the researcher enaged in several dummy runs of how best to lift one's feet off the treadmill, a not-straightforward technique using both hands/arms and lifting the feet from the revolving surface. Only when the participant was completely comfortable with the technique did the researcher then go on to secure written consent. He continued a dialogue with the participant throughout the exercise to ensure the welfare of the participant. This is a clear example of treating informed consent as a process and not a tick-box event. This model of good practice, it should be noted, also had the effect of giving maximal data, too – since the participant felt assured that he was well prepared in relation to the need to lift himself off the treadmill without fear of being ejected at velocity.

Written consent can serve to protect subjects as well as investigators. For researchers, a written record serves as proof that some attention has been paid to the interests of the subjects, and may in fact serve as defence in case of litigation. In addition to providing proof that ethical issues have been considered, written consent is superior to oral consent in that the form itself can be used as an explanatory tool and as a reference document in the communication process between researchers and subjects.

When there are doubts about the literacy level of subjects, however, oral information should supplement proxy written consent. Also, presenting information orally as well as in written form may have the advantage of prompting subjects to ask relevant questions. Witnessed consent may be particularly useful when subjects are elderly or have intellectual or cultural difficulties in speech or comprehension. In these cases, an independent person, such as a nurse or a religious leader, signs a document stating that the witness was present when the investigator explained the project to the potential subject, and that, in the opinion of the witness, consent was given freely and with understanding.

Finally, a consent form should not include language that absolves the researcher from blame, or any other waiver of legal rights releasing, or appearing to release anyone from liability (Liehmon, 1979; Veatch, 1989: 166). In any event, it is unlikely that such waivers would provide legal protection to researchers or institutions. The consent form should conclude with a statement that the subject has read the document and understands it, and should provide space underneath for his/her signature and the date. Space should also be provided for signatures of the researcher and an independent witness. Informed consent should be given on a written document.

Informed consent: some closing remarks

There are those who think that informed consent is a necessary condition of ethically defensible research. And there are those who think it is a sufficient condition of ethically defensible research. Neither position, as we have seen, is necessarily true. In this section we offer some closing remarks on the nature and importance of informed consent, which summarise what we have said thus far and attempt to situate this most important concept in research ethics in a more context-respectful light.

First, there will be occasions, despite their infrequency, where it is both necessary and justifiable to eschew the guidance we have given above and the very general obligation to gain informed consent. This, at least in part, is an acknowledgement of those, including O'Neill (2003), who claim *not* to use informed consent as an absolute and exceptionless principle. This may be under conditions of justified covert research (see Chapter 7) and where individual autonomy is not recognised as the most important norm as in cases of transcultural research and no significant harm is foreseen (see Chapter 9).

In contrast, the vast majority of research with human participants and subjects will entail the gaining of informed consent. This will typically entail consideration of the complex issues of competence and voluntariness we have set out above. Equally, it will render to the participant/subject all relevant knowledge and understanding to make the decision, and seek authorisation for it. It will assure participants and subjects to the appropriate degree that anonymity and confidentiality will be upheld. In order to effect this in an acceptable manner, it will involve a time-period relevant to the parameters of the research. With captive or vulnerable populations this will typically require some cooling-off period to avoid any possibility of coercion brought about by too swift a decision requirement. Moreover, where participation is extended over time it is good to revisit the participant with the issue of their desire to continue so as to reinforce the respect properly owed to them and to allow for discussion of ways in which the consent may have been given under conditions of incomplete knowledge, which might invalidate it. It also conforms to the general approach taken here, that informed consent be viewed as a process and not as a mere one-off, tick-box, externally imposed event.

Conclusion: a checklist for informed consent

This checklist is intended to help researchers meet their obligations to participants and subjects as well as the requirements of research ethics committee. It is not designed to replace the need to think through these issues carefully in the individual contexts of research across the spectrum of exercise, health and sports sciences. Moreover, it is vital that researchers also consider the local, regional or national requirements pertaining to informed consent as appropriate. Notwithstanding these disclaimers then, it will be helpful for researchers to cover the points listed below:

1 Ensure that you get voluntary, written, first-person informed consent.
2 Check institutional or legal guidelines about parental consent, and about obtaining a child's assent. In the case of using children as research subjects, you should obtain the necessary parental consent, and the child's assent.
3 When using vulnerable populations (e.g. the aged, wards of the state or other agencies), you should check that they comply with any ethical requirements specific to that group. For example, you may need witnessed consent for cognitively impaired subjects.
4 Satisfy yourself that subjects understand the nature of the project, including any risks or potential benefits. Describing the project to them verbally will often assist in this process.
5 Explain to subjects that they are free to ask questions at any time, and that they can withdraw from the project whenever they want to without threat of sanction.
6 Make sure that no coercion or undue influence occurs during the recruitment process. Satisfy yourself that any payments or inducements offered to subjects do not adversely influence their ability to make an informed assessment of the risks and benefits of participation.
7 Allow subjects a 'cooling off' period to consider their participation (the time between reading the form and actually agreeing to take part).
8 Assess the risk of physical, psychological or social harm to participants/subjects and make this clear to them.
9 Provide medical or other appropriate back-up in the event of any potential harm in the categories mentioned above.
10 Provide healthcare or other screening, as appropriate.

11 Assess the impact of any cultural and/or gender-specific issues that may pertain to your subjects, and/or the dissemination of your findings.
12 Provide adequate assurances regarding privacy, confidentiality, anonymity, and how you will securely store and treat your data, and then make sure you keep your promises to participants/subjects.
13 If your study involves deception, justify this with considerable care and indicate how you will debrief the subjects about the deception.
14 Put measures in place to provide subjects with appropriate feedback/information on completion of the project.

Adhering to these general prescriptions will not ensure that the research is itself ethical, nor will your research will necessarily move through IRB/REC approval without problems. It should, however, ensure that you cover the most basic considerations of ethically defensible research with particular relevance to the process of informed consent.

5   Whose datum is it anyway?

Anonymity, confidentiality and privacy

Conditions of anonymity, confidentiality and privacy are included in every informed consent form. Their presence is widely thought essential to protect subjects from harm, specifically with regard to preventing the dissemination of sensitive, attributable information. This chapter examines the soundness of reasons for the inclusion of these conditions in systems of research ethics, but also urges researchers critically to consider the particular meanings and purposes of the concepts as they are applied in a range of research contexts. As a general norm, confidentiality, for example, is at odds with the idea that research is to be disseminated and generalised. Nevertheless, there are situations where confidentiality is required, for instance in focus group work, or in health-care situations and in consultancy contexts.

Anonymity and identification are important issues, particularly in qualitative work, where 'rich' data or 'thick' description is necessary in order to make the research meaningful to the reader. Yet these matters, with implications for contextualisation and identification of individuals, are not simply to be set in the context of the individual researcher toiling away conscientiously. Almost all human participant/subject research takes place in some institutional context. Institutions provide the organisational base for research (including the researcher, the laboratory, leisure centre, sports club or hospital) and provide arenas in which research participants may be approached, recruited, observed and studied. Institutions too have responsibility for activities carried out in their name and obligations towards those who use their services and facilities. Institutions may thus have a corporate liability for the activities of researchers and the consequences of their actions. Some research carries genuine hazards and all human subject research entails some cost. These institutions therefore have an obligation to ensure that there are appropriate governance arrangements in place to protect the interests of all concerned. As part of that process, institutions are obliged to comply with the requirements of data protection legislation. As with all relationships between practitioners and institutions, this gives rise to certain tensions. It is the aim of this chapter to explore both the individual and institutional dimensions of the need to consider anonymity, confidentiality and privacy in the manifold aspects of the research process.

What's mine is mine: what ought respecting privacy to entail?

Confidentiality and anonymity may appear to some to be an obsession with Research Ethics Committees (RECs) and more generally in society. The UK popular press is full of stories about the Beckhams and Blairs and the revelations from nannies, au pairs and even art teachers in public schools. Some countries, for example France, have privacy laws, and campaigners have pressed for similar legislation in the UK, so far without success. Since 1970 Article 9 of the French Civil Code has provided that 'everyone has the right to respect for his or her private life'. A person's private life includes:

> his or her love life, friendships, family circumstances, leisure activities, political opinions, trade union or religious affiliation and state of health. In general, the right to privacy entitles anyone, irrespective of rank, birth, fortune or present or future office, to oppose the dissemination of his or her picture – an attribute of personality – without the express permission of the person concerned.
>
> (Embassy of France in the US, 2005)

While the French laws seek to protect the privacy of individuals, other countries have enacted legislation that significantly reduces the rights of the individual to privacy, as for example in the USA, where the so-called Patriot Act greatly increased the ability of government, among other things, to monitor private communications between individuals, through telephone tapping and electronic intercepts. In the UK the Data Protection Act was introduced to provide some regulation over the processing of personal information but its misapplication has been blamed for serious failures in police intelligence, which may have contributed to the deaths of two young children (Batty, 2003). At a more trivial level, it seems to be impossible to speak to any organisation about one's own affairs without first having to recite one's address, phone number, date of birth and mother's maiden name, all in the name of (supposedly) complying with the Act. In the context of research ethics, no researcher intending to collect personal data of any sort can ignore the issues of anonymity, confidentiality and privacy.

Application forms for RECs/IRBs invariably include sections concerning these issues; information sheets for participants will be expected to cover the question of anonymity and confidentiality, and consent forms will frequently seek explicit consent from participants for the handling of personal information and its disclosure to others involved in the research. Yet this norm stands in sharp relief, for example, with the position stated in a recent Editorial of the *British Medical Journal*:

> Some of the criticism of research ethics committees has focused on

issues for which they can bear no responsibility, such as the interpretation of the Data Protection Act.

(Ashcroft *et al.*, 2005: 557)

It is worth asking what, for many, will be taken for granted: precisely why is there such sensitivity toward personal data? To understand what is behind concerns about anonymity and confidentiality we must first explore the relationship between personal information, its value and impact, and the integrity of the self, as this relates to the concept of privacy. The ability to retain the right to choose what information to divulge or disclose to others, and what to retain to ourselves as privileged is an essential element of selfhood or personhood. Discovery of the ability not to reveal information, and even to lie, is a crucial stage in a child's development, as it marks the beginning of the development of the individual, private self. The ability to construct boundaries around our selves plays an important part in defining the difference between ourselves and others. Imagine, for example, that others had, as in a science fiction scenario, the ability to see inside our heads and read our minds. The result would be severely to destabilise the sense of self, and the belief that others can read our thoughts and manipulate our minds is a type of psychosis.

The removal of privacy, as happens in imprisonment, is seen as a punishment. In the eighteenth century the English utilitarian philosopher Bentham designed the Panopticon as a model prison in which 'the more constantly the persons to be inspected are under the eyes of the persons who should inspect them, the more perfectly will the purpose of the establishment have been attained'. This would be the case:

No matter how different, or even opposite the purpose: whether it be that of punishing the incorrigible, guarding the insane, reforming the vicious, confining the suspected, employing the idle, maintaining the helpless, curing the sick, instructing the willing in any branch of industry, or training the rising race in the path of education: in a word, whether it be applied to the purposes of perpetual prisons in the room of death, or prisons for confinement before trial, or penitentiary-houses, or houses of correction, or work-houses, or manufactories, or mad-houses, or hospitals, or schools.

(Bentham, 1995)

Foucault argues that 'the major effect of the Panopticon [is] to induce in the inmate a state of conscious and permanent visibility that assures the automatic functioning of power' (1995). In the context of health care, Girard (1988) talks about the elicitation of private information without sound justification as a form of sadism and an ontological assault. Thus invasion of privacy or the removal of privacy is no trivial matter, but may have a significant impact on the well-being of the person in question.

Can we be more specific than this? Parent (1983: 271–5) offers a critique of three conceptions of privacy that exist in ethical and jurisprudential writing:

1   privacy as being let alone;
2   privacy as autonomy;
3   Privacy as limitation on access to the self.

Each of these three conceptions has much to recommend it. Parent (1983) points out that were one to suffer innumerable blows to the head or be insulted from night to noon, the correct appeal would not simply be an appeal to privacy, but rather stronger, to concepts like force, harm or violence. Simply being let alone, then, does not capture what privacy depicts and, in the contexts of research, the notion of consent being denied seems to do the work that rights to privacy might entail. Second, although it is commonly the case that we think of privacy as control over significant personal matters, this conception fails to account for the person who divulges all sorts of intimate data about themselves; here the issue is one of a person who relinquishes their privacy while retaining control. And nothing seems wrong with this: indeed, often research with consent does not respect privacy in this sense of controlling when and who gets access to our privacy. There is something contradictory, then, about this conception. Closer, for our purposes, to understanding privacy as applied to research is the idea of limiting access to the self. But in this case we are left wondering precisely what limitations are intended; it might be thought that this implies some spatial characteristic like proximity. A paradigm of such a case would be when people seek court orders against stalkers. Can this really apply meaningfully to research situations where privacy of a different kind is in mind? What then is this privacy, and why is it thought to be so important?

Parent's positive account is this:

> Privacy is the condition of not having undocumented personal knowledge about one possessed by others [and that] . . . personal information consists of facts which most persons in a given society chose not to reveal about themselves . . . or of facts about which a particular individual is acutely sensitive and which he [sic] therefore does not choose to reveal about himself, even though most people do not care if these same facts are widely known about themselves.
>
> (Parent, 1983: 269–70)

Essentially, then, privacy refers to the ability to keep to ourselves information about ourselves that we choose not to disclose to others. This may relate to thoughts, opinions and feelings about anything, such as one's sexual preferences, the state of one's bank balance, or one's voting intentions. It is not just bad manners to pry into people's affairs, it may actually threaten a person's sense of self and security to feel that others have access to such information, regardless of the purposes for which they seek the information. A person's privacy is diminished exactly to the degree that others possess this kind of knowledge about him. The ability of others to obtain private information about us may also give them power over us, to do us harm, as for example in the case of Winston's experience with rats in Room 101 in George Orwell's *Nineteen Eighty-four* (2000 [1949]), or more recently, Cayce Pollard's phobia about the Michelin Man in William Gibson's *Pattern Recognition* (2003). The latter is a particularly telling example as the information was obtained from records stolen from the office of Pollard's psychotherapist. It is a warning, especially to those who work with sensitive data.

In an elite sporting context it is easy to imagine how information about a mental or physical frailty of an athlete or sportsman might give an advantage to a rival. Imagine how a sports psychologist working with batsmen in baseball or cricket, might give one access to their particular problems with a certain type of pitch or delivery. Or consider information about an elite distance runner who hated to run in the pack and ran best when heading the race with no-one around them. What about a dependency on prescription analgesics which were not performance enhancing but were enough to sully the reputation of a football player? One might expect that such information should not be leaked, not merely to other competitors but to anyone, even when the consultancy had ended.

In addition to the privacy of information in the more typical sense, contemporary society generally places value on the privacy of the body. This is perhaps more of a social construct than a deep-seated feature of our self-identity, because there have been times, and there are societies today, where the body and its functions were and are more public. Elias (1978), for example, describes how, since the eleventh century, the body has been 'privatised' and many of its functions made taboo.

The point about private information is *not* that no-one else may ever have access to it (although for some people, for some information, this may be true), but that the person to whom it is private retains control over its disclosure. One may choose (or be compelled) to disclose certain things to certain people in whom one places trust. In a personal relationship one may share personal information because this in some way strengthens the relationship. You share your deepest emotions with your lover because, given that our individual personal privacy is what keeps us separate and differentiated from others, you wish to be closer to your lover, to reduce or remove the barriers or boundaries that separate you, to unite you in your relationship. Members of the Catholic religion may confess what they would describe as their sins in order to maintain their relationship with the Church and their God. With friends or colleagues one may share hopes, fears, ambitions and so on, in the interest of strengthening the bonds of friendship or creating a better team.

Or, more instrumentally or prudentially, one may disclose intimate and personal information to a doctor, a solicitor, a bank manager or an accountant, because they cannot work effectively on one's behalf unless this is done. But whereas in the context of a love affair we may disclose completely, absolutely, as proof of the strength of our love for and trust in the other, in professional and service relationships we disclose within a structure of rules, and these rules are set by the context. So, to take an example from Weinberg, it is possible to be nude in front of others without embarrassment as long as we adhere to the rules appropriately in the context. Being naked in a nudist camp is acceptable, but walking in the nude from Land's End to John O'Groats (i.e. the length of the UK) apparently is not (see BBC, 2004).

The story of Stephen Gough, who set out to challenge the attitude of society to the human body, also illustrates the point that disclosure is not always welcomed by others. Revealing that which society prefers to keep concealed can provoke censure and sanctions: Gough took seven months to complete his trek from Cornwall to Scotland, in part because of the number of times he was arrested and imprisoned following complaints from members of the public. Being naked in the changing rooms and the showers at the sports facility, or sharing a bath with someone of the same sex is commonplace after a rugby match. But it is less likely that two members of the same rugby team sharing a hotel room on tour would be happy to share a bath in their hotel bathroom, even if they regularly shared an ice bath after the match. And just as public nudity is bound by rules in context, we disclose personal information to the doctor or solicitor in a context that is also informed by rules, explicit or implicit.

One of the possible consequences of unwanted disclosure of personal information, whether about our thoughts, feelings, actions or the appearance of our bodies, is embarrassment or shame. Privacy is about not disclosing to people certain information about ourselves, and being obliged to give information that we would not otherwise wish to disclose reveals something about us that we would prefer to remain hidden. As Sartre (2003) suggests, when we are caught performing a disreputable act – he suggests peeping through a keyhole or making a rude gesture – we feel shame not because of the act itself but because we have revealed to the person who catches us, something about the kind of person we really are.

If someone seeks legal representation because they have been caught stealing they will typically reveal to the solicitor that they are a dishonest person, and that, at least for most people, is shameful. A visit to the sexually transmitted disease clinic to investigate a urethral discharge reveals to the staff that the patient has had sex with someone who has gonorrhoea or some such. Because of they way the body has become privatised, as Elias argues, even admitting the existence of a problem with bladder or bowel functions may cause feelings of embarrassment or shame, even though concealing symptoms may increase the probability of serious illness or even death from bowel cancer, for example. In discussing our bodily functions we are revealed as the kind of person who cannot manage their body in the way that society expects.

We disclose these embarrassing circumstances to our doctors or lawyers on the assumption that, in their professional roles, they will be non-judgemental. We do not expect to be given a lecture on morality by these people, although some professional advice about my future conduct may well be expected. But we properly expect our doctor to pronounce on the condition of our health without offering a critique of our character. We give an extended discussion of privacy as it relates to qualitative research in Chapter 7.

Research participants/subjects disclose personal information in these professional circumstances and rule-limited settings with two provisos: that they give their consent and that they are assured of confidentiality. Despite the lengthy treatment of informed consent in Chapter 4 it may be worth rehearsing a few salient points here in the context of anonymity, confidentiality and privacy, for they are clearly supposed to be linked.

The contemporary view of consent in this context means that disclosure is voluntary, where the option of not disclosing is present. Of course, we may feel that in reality we have little choice. If we withhold essential information from a professional we jeopardise our chances of success in the enterprise for which we have consulted them, while in our personal relationships to be less than frank and open with lovers or friends exposes us to the risk that the relationship will fail.

Our access or entry to certain events or situations may be conditional on our consent to a certain level of disclosure as, for example, when we submit to a drug-testing regime as a requirement for competing in athletics. But we have the existential choice, nevertheless, as to whether we disclose or not.

How far ought researchers to go to keep confidences confidential?

Confidentiality provides what might be thought of as an extension of the boundaries of the self. Research participants or subjects are typically prepared to disclose some information, even of a personal nature, but only on the basis that they can rely on the confidence of researchers to hold the information in trust and *in that confidence*, not to further disclose without their permission and agreement. Thus participants or subjects retain control over access to personal information even though they have disclosed it. It will be useful to consider some realistic though hypothetical examples to illustrate these points.

A researcher began collecting longitudinal data (collected over a period over five years) on the lifestyles of elite sportspersons with respect to casual drug habits. The data were kept in locked files in a locked office to which few people had access. A few years into the research a politically conservative chief executive officer (CEO) of the sports governing body was appointed. A request was made to the CEO by a local police detective who suspected that the researcher's files might help him track down potential drug dealers.

Having been granted a search warrant, the police visited the researcher at his desk and seized the files. This enabled access to a wide range of personal, confidential data. Who could foresee such a scenario? Would it not be unreasonable to have demanded the researcher to have done more? What are the limits of confidentiality between researcher, subject and other institutions? What could or ought the researcher do or have done? One course of action which it is reasonable to expect of researchers, especially so in the light of sensitive data, is for the researcher to consider themselves under a duty to keep separate the schedule of anonymous identifiers of research participants/subjects and to store it in a place that is not readily accessible. This is the least that one might expect from the researcher. The identifiers must not be kept on the same files, or in the same folders, or even on the same computer as the schedule which might identify them.

Some key questions arise from this scenario then are as follows:

1   Precisely how and where do researchers record data?
2   What systems will be used for identifying characteristics?
3   How and where is the data stored?
4   Who has access to the data?
5   How long is the data held for?

While the first four questions have arisen in the discussion and require no further comment it is worth making an observation on the holding of data. Typically, one can make a somewhat trite and generalised observation here: do not hold data longer than is necessary; or destroy data when it is no longer of use to the research. Of course the difficulty is to know precisely *when* such time has arrived. In the cases of research degree students, it is clear that the need to hold on to the data clearly extends to the length of the process, at least until the award of the relevant degree. And it is reasonable to assume, with pressures to publish such as they are, that this time period extends for some years after this. Professional organisations and research codes of conduct give differing advice. And why should we expect homogeneity when we consider the needs and processes of, for example, archival research, focus group work, random clinical trials? One norm, which has been found in many cases, is that of five years after data has been collected. But no particular weight can be assigned to this. At least it may set a line, however arbitrary, that the researcher must respect and if necessary return to the IRB or REC to gain an extension. This at least binds the researcher to the commitment of the informed consent process, that the data will be destroyed at the earliest relevant date. On the other hand it could be argued that premature destruction of data, collected at some expense, is itself immoral. Some research councils are encouraging the archiving of qualitative data as this may provide a valuable long-term and historical resource. Similarly, in medical research, tissue samples may be collected and held in banks for future research in studies and for purposes that have not yet been imagined.

Provided proper consent is obtained, and the conditions of storage and future use are made clear at the time, there may be a case for certain kinds of data to be stored indefinitely.

A final health warning is required by way of summary. Researchers must be careful in the way in which they pose the issues of confidentiality. Too often one sees on IRBs/RECs cases where researchers in a cavalier way simply assert that privacy and confidentiality will be absolutely preserved. While we have shown how this can be undone by a lack of thought in the collection and presenting of research, we are obliged to note that researchers do not have legal authority to withhold data in cases of criminal action. If the law forces us, we must disclose (on pain of becoming a research 'martyr'). Protest about the protection of participants or subjects as one may, disrespect of the judge and their court may cost researchers a custodial sentence.

Consider another case, which involves role conflict. Imagine you are a physiotherapist who has been performing strength evaluations over the last five years as part of a research-based consultancy programme with a sports national governing body. You hope to publish the data to support a new massage-therapy technique with over-use soft-tissue injuries. The governing body which funds your work is about to review its funding in relation to cutbacks in its overall budget. There is a feeling that certain 'senior' athletes are carrying career-threatening injuries and will not be able to recover before the next Olympics. In particular, one athlete appears to have had a recurrent injury and is thought to have a structural weakness. The governing body wants access to her data over the last five years to see if there is a pattern of injury, which it will use as a basis to decide whether its funding is continued or withdrawn.

The most general questions that arises in this context are:

1   What happens when research norms and contract obligations collide?
2   What obligations are owed to the subjects extend over time?
3   How ought the researcher to cater for non-immediate considerations?

If the capture of the data has adhered to the norms above, then at least if seizure of the files happens the code will not have been accessed, and the data will remain suitably unidentifiable. Given that the example utilises personal data, participants/subjects have a right to expect that the data has been written up appropriately (avoiding the specification of name, location, special circumstances, ethnicity, etc.) and stored in an appropriately safe place. In addition, and in proportion to the perceived sensitivity or potential sensitivity of the data, any special characteristics of participants/subjects must be altered, and consideration given to the nature of alteration, especially where the research may become public. Consideration ought also to be given as to whether the research should be made public, however publishable it might be.

Researchers must make clear at the outset of externally funded research issues pertaining to the ownership of the data. This can help to forestall problems at a later date. By thinking through as carefully as is possible the potential scenarios one can avoid many of the misfortunes of identification of research participants. Of course, this will not always be possible. If there are potential ambiguities in anonymity, confidentiality or privacy, then it may well be appropriate not to raise the expectations of the researched at the outset of the research. Then this informed consent will entail a realistic recognition of whether the data might be compromised, leaked or simply published, and the participant then knowingly offers or withholds their consent. Equally, if circumstances alter during the course of the research in relation to these issues, then respecting consent as a process entails that researchers must go back and negotiate consent for the data. Equally, they ought to destroy previous data collected if it is the wish of the participant/subject.

Anonymised data collection and reporting – a gold standard?

Data that is truly anonymous is not, as the Medical Research Council (MRC) argues, 'personal', as it cannot be associated with any individual. Truly anonymised data cannot therefore be said to breach privacy or confidentiality. A good example of this comes from the mid-1990s, with the unlinked, anonymised HIV screening programme in England and Wales (Banatvala, 1995). In order to monitor the prevalence of HIV many thousands of blood samples were tested. These samples came from people who had entered the health-care system for some other reason, for example attending ante-natal clinics, and samples of blood had all identifying labels removed and were then tested for HIV. Such testing of course offers no benefit to the person tested as individuals have no way of obtaining the results of their test. The information simply gave an indication of changes in the prevalence of the virus in various groups in the population. Anonymised testing of this kind has the advantage that it carries no risk for the patient. Many people would have been reluctant to be tested on a named basis as at that time the mere fact of having been tested could prove problematic for life insurance, for example. One can imagine that similar anonymisation of athletes for various substances might give a more accurate indication of the prevalence of use of various stimulants or performance aids, without the athletes being at risk of detection. Even the remotest possibility of failures of anonymity would mean that few would entertain participation in such tests.

The challenge, of course, is to ensure genuine anonymity. In a theoretical sense there may no longer be any such thing as anonymised samples: all of the blood samples tested in the HIV prevalence study could be identified by DNA matching if a matching sample could be found. With increasing numbers of people having their DNA recorded for one reason or another, and with various proposals for a national DNA database, true anonymity may be a thing of the past. Countries such as Iceland and Estonia have already begun to construct a national database, while in the UK the police database holds DNA records for almost 3 million people and the inventor of the technology, Sir Alec Jeffries, has argued for a complete, population-wide database (Wellcome Trust, 2004).

Not all personal data includes tissue samples, and even for those that do, DNA matching is probably not a serious issue at present, so let us assume that data could be anonymised. The MRC in the UK has issued guidelines on the processing of personal information for research that can serve as a model for any discussion in this area. Apart from information that is plainly identifiable, the MRC differentiates between three categories of data: coded data; anonymised linked data; and anonymised unlinked data.

1   Coded data includes information from which people could be identified, but obvious identifiers such as names will be replaced with a code. The code will be linked to a key, which will be held by the researchers but stored separately so that no-one could easily gain unauthorised access.
2   Anonymised linked data is similar to coded data, but it is anonymised to the researchers. For example, a hospital might extract a data set from patient records, create a numbered key, remove personal identifiers and replace them with the code number and pass the data on to the research team in this form.
3   Anonymised unlinked data is data from which identifiers have been removed with no means of restoring the link. Interestingly, the MRC say that unlinked data has nothing in it 'that has reasonable potential' to allow the identification of the individual, which rather leaves open the question of what would count as reasonable.

Finally, the MRC state that as a minimum such data must not include:

*   name, address, phone/fax number
*   email address, full postcode
*   NHS number or any other identifying reference number
*   photograph, or names of relatives.

The MRC acknowledges that, even with these precautions, there is the potential to deduce the identity of a research participant. They identify the most problematic data items as:

*   rare disease or treatment, especially if an easily noticed illness/disability is involved
*   partial postcode, or partial address
*   place of treatment or health professional responsible for care
*   rare occupation or place of work
*   combinations of birth date, ethnicity, place of birth and date of death.

Recent discussion, in the light of the UK Data Protection Act, has focused on whether RECs are being too defensive, even zealous, in their interpretation of the Act with respect to anonymised data. Walley (2006) has gone so far as to argue that the request for direct consent for routinely collected data can seriously hamper, for example, epidemiological health research, by making it expensive and – where it is not sought – by making the data less useful. This claim is supported by his contention, after Verity and Nicholl (2002), that the kinds of data required for epidemiological research are thin when compared with intervention research in health and medicine. It is unclear whether this utilitarian justification for access to data not directly consented for is sufficient given the concerns over privacy of data itself. He argues that recent research gives support (Robling *et al.*, 2004; Iversen *et al.*, 2006) to the need for much greater communication with the public to determine whether research ethics demands have run too far ahead of the public's will in such matters.

Preserving anonymity might be both natural and straightforward in random clinical trials. It is far less easy in the collection and analysis of rich data that might emerge in qualitative research such as in focus groups or group interviews. Here anonymity is simply an unrealistic goal and statements to the effect of preserving it should not appear on any informed consent form or verbal negotiation. There is thus no gold standard for research in these matters. In every case there must be the sensitivity and sensible application of the very general norms.

It is easy to see how such information could lead to an individual, even when data has supposedly been anonymised and unlinked: if one lives in a small area and has some unique characteristic one may be easily recognised, a situation that might be described as the 'only black African in the village' factor. In a sporting context it may be that very few people fit a particular profile, of perhaps being an Olympic champion, in an event such as the men's hurdles, and living in Cardiff.

When collecting data by questionnaire, for example, there is a tendency to take down as much demographic data as one can in a rather unplanned manner. Identification of subjects can arise when – with smaller data sets especially – there are only so many men of a given ethnicity and a given age within an organisation. Yet researchers should frequently ask themselves whether all demographic data is essential to answering the questions set out in the research design. Equally, when presenting data, particularly in public forums such as contract research reports, scientific journal articles, conference presentations or indeed lectures, researchers should think hard about the categories in which data about individuals or groups is presented, so that they do not become so specialised or discrete that participants or subjects can be identified.

The issue of using focus groups on sensitive subjects has been identified as potentially problematic (Morgan and Kreuger, 1993; Zeller, 1993; Bringer *et al.*, 2002). One recent example in the literature, which pertains to the collection of data from swimming coaches regarding issues of harassment and abuse (Bringer, 2002), is a model of good practice. Following identification of leakage of extremely sensitive and potentially illegal activity, the university REC inquired how confidentiality would be handled in the research. The researcher's response was to recognise the lack of control over the data and the situation. In response she adopted the following strategy:

- all participants were discouraged from making inappropriate disclosures
- all participants used aliases to avoid identification of particular persons in the discussion
- all participants signed a confidentiality agreement separate to the informed consent form
- participants were reminded at the beginning of the focus groups about the need to avoid inappropriate disclosure
- participants were reminded that they had a right to remain silent should they so wish.

It is important to remember that, in the informed consent process, participants and subjects will have been promised confidentiality and/or anonymity to an appropriate degree. Failing to live up to that promise because of planning failure is both poor research and ethically culpable.

The benefits and harms associated with anonymity, privacy and confidentiality

Having sketched out some of the groundwork for the notions of anonymity, confidentiality and privacy we can turn now to a consideration of the goods, wrongs and harms that may be associated with these concepts. Let us assume that, other things being equal, privacy and respectful confidentiality are goods, for the reasons suggested above. Are invasions of privacy and breaches of confidence harmful and are we wronged by them?

It is important to distinguish between being wronged and being harmed. A failure to respect a person's privacy or to keep a confidence is a failure to respect the person and is thus a moral wrong, something we ought not to do and for which we would be thought blameworthy. Feinberg, for example, defines a wrong as an act, performed with an appropriate type of fault, that violates the rights of another without excuse or justification (Stewart, 2002). And it is worth noting that, for most people, wrongs and harms can to some extent be independent of each other: one can for instance be wronged without being harmed. The final report of the Advisory Committee on Human Radiation Experiments, set up in 1994 by the US Department of Energy, to investigate research into the effects of radiation conducted between the 1940s and the 1970s, notes that:

The entire Committee believes that people who were used as research subjects without their consent were wronged even if they were not harmed. Although it is surely worse, from an ethical standpoint, to have been both harmed and wronged than to have been used as an unwitting subject of experiments and suffered no harm, it is still a moral wrong to use people as a mere means.

(ACHRE, n.d.)

In a similar vein, the Draft Report of the US National Bioethics Advisory Commission argues that:

In addition to harms, at least narrowly construed, there are wrongs to individuals and groups, for example, in the violation of rights such as a right to privacy. Not every wrong, such as an unjustified breach of privacy, is itself a harm or even causes a harm. For instance, if someone enters our house and rummages through our personal possessions, but takes nothing and leaves everything exactly as it was before so that we don't know that anything occurred, it is appropriate to say that we have been wronged, because our right to privacy was violated, even though no harm occurred. People may be harmed without being wronged and wronged without being harmed. In short, an ethical framework needs the concept of wrongs as well as the concept of harms.

(NBAC, 1999: 4)

So, by this analysis, even if the victim has no knowledge that his or her privacy has been invaded or confidentiality breached, he or she has been wronged. Invasions of privacy and breaches of confidence are thus simply wrongs, regardless of the consequences. But what if such invasions or breaches were accidental? What part does intention play? If the breach were completely accidental, indeed, if I became the unwilling recipient of private information about you, I might well be thought to be blameless but you might nevertheless feel wronged. And what, then, if I knowingly, deliberately, pry into your affairs without your knowledge, or disclose information that I was given in confidence, will this be a wrong regardless of the intention? If, for example, as your friend, I suspect you may have made some unwise financial decisions, and I take it upon myself to go through your private papers without your knowledge, so that I can take some action on your behalf that saves you from financial ruin, is this as bad as, for example, sneaking a look at your pay slip so that I can negotiate my own salary increase from a stronger position?

From a utilitarian perspective it is tempting to say that breaches of privacy or confidentiality should be judged as blameworthy or praiseworthy on the basis of the consequences. There are close similarities here with lying and promise-keeping – if we have undertaken to keep something confidential breaching that confidence is a form of lying or a breach of a promise. I said I would keep the information confidential but I lied – I have now passed it on to several others. Bentham says: 'Falsehood, taken by itself, consider it as not being accompanied by any other material circumstances, nor therefore productive of any material effects, can never, upon the principle of utility, constitute any offence at all' (Bentham in Bok, 1978b). Martin Luther apparently said 'What harm would it do, if a man told a good strong lie for the sake of the good and for the Christian church . . . a lie out of necessity, a useful lie, a helpful lie, such lies would not be against God, he would accept them.'

So, for these authors, the degree of wrong depends very much on the consequence. There is a longer heritage of this idea, back to Plato, as the 'noble lie'. A counter-argument of course might be that, to take Luther's example, 'a good strong lie' is an oxymoron, a lie cannot be good, and lies told about the Church (or any other institution) must necessarily weaken it rather than be helpful, simply because of the dishonesty. If, as a representative of an institution, I lie to you, with the supposed intention of raising your estimation of the institution, but you find out that I have lied to you about it, then you may form the general opinion that the type of people associated with the institution are those who are dishonest, and so you may want nothing to do with it.

We made the distinction earlier between being wronged and being harmed. What is required for a harm to occur? Is the mere fact of being wronged a harm in itself or must there be adverse consequences? It is generally accepted that to be harmed is to have one's interests adversely affected. Thus we may be wronged without necessarily being harmed, and we may be harmed without knowing that we have been harmed. Being wronged may of course advance our interests, in that we may benefit from receiving some redress, or benefiting from the sympathy and consideration of others who perceive the harm and seek to offer some remedy.

How we view the nature of harm depends also on how we understand the relationship between harm and suffering. We may suffer no more than annoyance that our privacy has been invaded or a confidence breached. We may experience embarrassment or shame at being found out, as for example if our attendance at the sexually transmitted illnesses clinic is revealed to others, particularly those whose esteem we value. But there may be actual, quantifiable damage, if, for example, disclosure of one's HIV positive status were to lead to social isolation, loss of a job or the inability to obtain life insurance.

As Bok (1978b) points out, fully appreciating the consequences of dishonesty, whether in breaking promises, lying or breaching a confidence, is difficult and is not just confined to the immediate effects. A friend may be saved from financial ruin by my dishonest actions, but at what price to the relationship and to my trustworthiness in future dealings? And for Bok there is a real sense that whatever the consequences for others, harm is incurred by the dishonest person, in terms of their self-respect and integrity.

Research involving human participation necessarily involves the disclosure of personal information and may involve significant invasion of privacy. We suggest that the analysis of truly anonymised data does not involve human participation in any meaningful way. As the MRC argues, it is not strictly speaking 'personal information' (MRC, 2000). But as long as actual individuals, identifiable as such, are involved, then disclosure is inevitable. Whether the study involves observation, interviews, questionnaires, interventions or any other type of data collection the researcher inevitably receives information about the participant.

Clearly some types of study require the disclosure of more personal, sensitive information than others. In-depth qualitative interviews about some very intimate experience may raise many difficult issues, as for example if a researcher investigating the experience of young athletes of coaching by adult instructors revealed evidence of abuse or improper relationships. Detailed investigations of training methods, nutritional supplements and other such interventions may reveal the use of prohibited substances. Physical testing, for example exercising to exhaustion, will reveal the abilities and limitations of an athlete, in ways that he or she may not wish to be exposed. The analysis of blood and other body fluids or tissue samples reveals information about the individual that may go well beyond the basic data that the participant expected to reveal. Even simple questionnaires or observation in public places represent an intrusion into people's lives.

Conclusion: anonymous, confidential, private (in context)

When considering this family of research ethics concerns, a key question for researchers then is whether their work involves the defensible collection of personal information. While research does necessarily require the disclosure of information, the necessary extent of that information is debatable. Researchers should always consider the virtue of parsimony and only collect data that can be justified as necessary to answer the research questions. When designing a study and developing the data set required for analysis, researchers should test every item of data against the question of what it is to be used for: if there is not a sound justification for its use to answer the research question then it should not be collected. This is scientifically sound as well as an ethical requirement.

The justification for disclosure of personal information in research must be considered in a very different context from disclosure in other settings. Given our earlier account of the importance of privacy for the maintenance of the self as distinctive and separate from others, the legitimate reasons why disclosure may be desirable or beneficial, and the nature and importance of confidentiality, the expectation that others may disclose personal information in the course of participating in research, must be supported by several considerations.

In other areas of our lives our decisions to disclose personal information are usually taken in the context of some relationship in which we perceive a benefit for ourselves or for the quality of the relationship from the disclosure.

We allow access to our private selves because to do so seems likely to further our interests in some way. However, it is usually the case that participants in research cannot assume that they will accrue any direct benefit from that research or from the disclosure that such participation requires. The study may fail to produce any beneficial results, or any beneficial results that do occur may not be directly relevant to any given individual who took part in the study, or may come too late for those individuals and so on. There is thus always the possibility of altruism in human participation – the participant may be sufficiently rewarded by the thought that his or her involvement helped to advance knowledge and might eventually benefit others.

For some people it is of course possible that there is some pleasure or satisfaction to be gained from involvement in research. We may feel some sense of reflected glory or self-importance from being part of a research study. Or it may be that there are actual benefits from involvement in a study. In the context of medical research it is frequently claimed that participants in trials make better progress with their health than do those not in the trial, regardless of which treatment they receive. This is said in part to be the result of the additional attention received, and the very thorough and rigorous adherence to treatment protocols and monitoring of vital signs and so on. We know of no studies currently to relate this to exercise or sports sciences, but it would seem plausible to imagine that athletes entering an experimental training regime or rehabilitation programme following injury might receive similar benefits. The challenge for researchers is, minimally, to develop and maintain respectful and responsible relations with the researched. Whether the failure to preserve anonymity, or confidentiality or privacy of data or identities is brought about by acts of commission or omission, researchers may be thought to be culpable. Therefore, they ought always to take well-planned steps to avoid improperly exploiting the willingness of people to participate in research or by failing to live up to the promises set out in the consent process.

6 Scientific misconduct

Authorship, plagiarism and fraud, and blowing the whistle on it

The slogan 'Publish or perish!', though melodramatic, sums up life for many academics from professors to research assistants. Academics are authors as a matter of necessity: appointment to a post, the successful completion of a probationary period in a new job, research income and promotion, all require evidence of published work. If there were any doubt as to the capacity of this trend to produce pernicious results, the words of Grinnell should be compulsory reading:

> Modern science in the United States finds itself in the midst of a crisis. The scope of this crisis encompasses the entire scientific enterprise from its mission to its funding to the conduct of individual scientists in laboratories. How can we expect policy makers and the public to understand and respond to these issues effectively if scientists cannot reach a consensus on the principles and practices that guide research? If we don't explain why ambiguity is inherent in the day-to-day practice of science, then we might find the practice of research restricted in ways that make creative insight far more difficult.
>
> (Grinnell, 1997: 192)

The trend, which emerged in the US, certainly has a more global reach now as research management and accountability have emerged and developed apace in universities.[1] And apart from the personal agenda of struggling researchers, scientific knowledge is by definition publicly verifiable: for many people new work does not count as a contribution to knowledge until it has been made public and subjected to independent scrutiny. This will usually be through the peer review process or, in the case of research degrees, by the examiners. Once work has passed the peer review process it can then be considered by a wider readership, who will also have their own views about its validity and importance. Considerable scorn is heaped upon the scientist who elects to give his findings their first public exposure through a press conference or by publication in the popular media. Publication in peer reviewed journals gives the reader some reassurance that others, expert in the field, have examined the author's work and found it convincing.

But if publication is a crucial step in the establishment of knowledge, it is also the area in which there are perhaps the greatest temptations for unscrupulous individuals to go astray. So important is publication for the rewards of academic status and financial gain that it would be surprising if there were not examples of dubious practice and dishonesty. However rigorous the process of examination and peer review, the only real assurance we have that work has been presented truthfully is the honesty and integrity of the author.

In this chapter we will review something of the history and nature of misconduct in research and discuss the ethical implications of authorship. Given the generally casuistical approach outlined in Chapter 2, our stance here will be broadly drawn from virtue ethics. The ethical requirements of authorship, in our view, are such that no amount of consideration of principles, duties or consequences will be sufficient on its own. In virtue ethics intention is all, and what is required of the author of research publications, we claim, is a deep-rooted understanding of the importance of integrity and the intention to be honest.

What is scientific misconduct?

Before delving in to the particular sins of scientists and scholars it is worth noting a more general account of what constitutes scientific misconduct. It is our assumption that, generally speaking, serious misconduct is a relatively rare occurrence. We address some spectacular exceptions to this norm, such as the fabrication of data and research (see 'Credit and other issues of multiple authorship', pp. 112–16 and 'Research fraud', pp. 120–2). Typically less worrying though probably more frequent examples of misconduct are represented by the varieties of plagiarism, which are given extended discussion (see 'Plagiarism', pp. 116–20).

We take from Grinnell (1997) a reasonably wide definition of research misconduct into which these prime examples fit. He observes the commonsensical point that few cases are simply 'black and white' such as outright lies (e.g. reporting experiments that never happened) or stealing (e.g. word-for-word plagiarism), yet if the research falls under the following criteria Grinnell suggests we can label it 'scientific misconduct' unambiguously:

1 The activities are not part of the normal practice of science.
2 A person's single action is sufficient to infer misconduct.
3 The intention to deceive is implicit in the action itself.

Grinnell goes on to problematise the designation of research misconduct when applied to individual scientists and scholars. He does so by drawing upon the autobiography of the biomedical researcher Levi-Montalcini (cited in Grinnell, 1997: 189) who wrote:

even though I possessed no proof in favour of the hypothesis, in my secret heart of hearts I was certain that the tumors that had been transplanted into the embryos would in fact stimulate fiber growth.

When this did not happen Levi-Montalcini wrote in a letter that this was:

the most severe blow to my enthusiasm that I could have ever suffered. . . . After suffering the brunt of the initial shock at these results, in a partially unconscious way I began to apply what Alexander Luria, the Russian neuropyschologist, has called 'the law of disregard of negative information . . . facts that fit into a preconceived hypothesis attract attention, are singled out, and remembered. Facts that are contrary to it are disregarded, treated as exception, and forgotten.

(Levi-Montalcini, 1998, cited in Grinnell, 1997: 189)

Cases such as these throw up the difficulty of separating ethical from psychological explanations and justifications. Clearly the 'law of disregard' does not happen at a conscious level. There is no active intention to deceive or mislead others, yet it should warn anyone who thinks that they are inured against culpable error simply armed with the shibboleth called the *scientific method* (see Toulmin, 2001: 83–101) or relevant research training. Science is and always will be an all-too-human affair. But there is another tension worth observing. This is between the ethical dimensions of research, and these are often combined with, or at least contributive to, epistemological ones. Sometimes naïve appeals to the duty of researchers to search for the truth (or truths for certain postmodern or post-structural researchers) fail to take account of the messiness of research. Grinnell quotes Jacob:

writing a paper is to substitute order for the disorder and agitation that animate life in the laboratory . . . to get some work accepted and a new way of thinking adopted, it is necessary to purify the research of all affective or irrational dross. To get rid of any personal scent, any human smell . . . to replace the real order of events and discoveries by what appears as the logical order, the one that should have been followed if the conclusions were known from the start.

From which he concludes:

In research papers, one finds only demonstrative research: the investigator's current thinking illustrated by successful and complete experiments stylised according to the expectations of the community about how data should be collected and presented. The research will be organized into a coherent story with the plot none other than *the scientific method*.

(Jacob, 1988: 318, cited in Grinnell, 1997: 191)

There is a difficulty, then, between issues of truthfulness and professionalism which belies the conceptions of both science and ethics in terms of universalistic rules for researchers and particularistic or casuistic applications of them. Grinnell observes that this ambiguity, which he believes is probably inherent in the processes of scientific and scholarly production will frustrate naïve principalists who simply demand that scientists are truthful and fair. What we shall attempt in the remainder of this chapter is a specification of the chief examples of research misconduct and how they are present in the different forms of scholarship in exercise, health and sports sciences.

Authorship and the virtues of authors

Thinking casually about the status of author, one might be forgiven for going no further than something like 'the person who writes the words on the page'. Consider then the following definitions from the *Shorter Oxford English Dictionary*:

> Author: The person who originates or gives existence to anything; he who gives rise to an action, event, circumstance or state of things; one who begets, a father; one who sets forth written statements, the writer or composer of a treatise or book. Authorship: the dignity of an author, literary origin or origination. Origination of an action, state of affairs etc.

As we can see from the definitions given above, authorship implies rather more than the person responsible for the appearance of words on a page. The cliché of the ecstatic audience, cheering and stamping their feet and crying 'Author, author!' reminds us that the author is much more than the scribe or transcriber, the secretarial hand that takes down the words of others. This is the person who 'originates or gives existence to' the work, the person who 'begets' it. 'Authorship' refers to 'the dignity of an author' and dignity is a distinctly moral concept. Authorship implies responsibility and accountability but it also brings with it any credit that may deserved, depending on the quality and importance of the work. As Hooey (2000: 6) says, credit and responsibility 'are the twin attributes of authorship'. A claim to authorship is a claim of ownership and, if it is a claim to be the originator, then it must also be a claim, at least to some extent, to originality. And thus claims of authorship carry with them a range of moral commitments which include but are not exhausted by the following: authenticity, honesty, integrity and truthfulness. These qualities are, of course, examples of the moral virtues, qualities which, we would argue, are necessary attributes of the researcher and the academic author.

Research and academic work are practices, using that term in the particular sense developed by MacIntyre:

any coherent and complex socially established cooperative human activity through which goods internal to that form of activity are realized in the course of trying to achieve those standards of excellence which are appropriate to, and partially definitive of, that form of activity, with the result that human powers to achieve excellence and human conceptions of the ends and goods involved are systematically extended.

(MacIntyre, 1984: 187)

In developing his account, MacIntyre draws attention to the different goods available as a result of engagement with a practice, goods which he characterises as being either internal or external to the practice. Internal goods are available only to those who engage in the practice, while external goods are the material rewards, of money and status, which may follow success in any occupation. Critically, for MacIntyre, entering a practice requires the possession of the moral virtues on the part of the practitioner, in particular the virtues of courage, honesty and justice. Importantly in the context of research and publishing, MacIntyre observes the dangers of the pursuit of external goods and the inevitability of the effacement of the virtues in consequence.

Sustaining virtues like integrity and honesty (let alone humility) in the face of the considerable pressures academics are placed under is no easy matter.

It would be inappropriate and sociologically naïve to place under the microscope only individuals concerned: clearly a fair evaluation of these difficulties and the persons involved must crucially bear witness to the prevailing ethos of research in a given university, or faculty, or even laboratory, as well as to national policies that drive the world of publishing. The power of authority figures to lay down the professional norms of natural and social scientists is not to be underestimated. Sometimes there is a near macho drive to publish outrageous quantities of research papers, which can do little but enlarge the ego of key personnel and simultaneously corrupt the initiates such as graduate students or research assistants in the process. Institutional policing may be necessary, but the promotion of better role-models, and greater attention being paid to the processes of research training and education as well will be more effective in the long term.

Credit and other issues of multiple authorship

When an individual works alone and is the sole author of a piece of work the question of attribution and origination is relatively straightforward. Trusting that the author is honest and did actually complete the work which he or she is reporting, then the one name appears on the resulting essay, report, dissertation or article. However, perhaps the majority of academic writing these days involves more than one author. Most of us work in departments, or research groups, or some other kind of team and we collaborate with colleagues in other institutions. This book is precisely such an example. Two of us are former colleagues, but all three work in different institutions, indeed now in different countries. The many people working on projects all naturally wish to have their contribution acknowledged, not just from vanity but because their very careers may depend upon getting their names on the right papers in the right journals. Security of tenure, promotion and future research income will all depend to some extent on the quantity and quality of publications a scholar has to his name.

The complexities of the situation are illustrated by Hooey (2000), who describes the publication of the historically momentous finding of the effect of pancreatic extract on diabetes in 1922. Hooey reports that:

> The authors were Banting, Best, Collip, Campbell and Fletcher. Notably missing was Macleod, who would, with Banting, receive the 1923 Nobel Prize for medicine and share his portion of the prize money with Collip, as Banting shared his with Best. Macleod and 3 others (Henderson, Fitzgerald and Graham) were thanked at the end of the paper for 'their hearty co-operation and kindly assistance and advice.' As Michael Bliss has entertainingly documented, the sometimes explosive disputes over the control of the research that led to the discovery of insulin and over who should take credit for it were legendary even at the time.
>
> (Hooey, 2000: 6)

The problem was that the members of the 1922 research team all contributed in different ways. According to Hooey:

> Banting is usually credited with persisting with the idea that the pancreas contained a substance that regulated blood sugar. Best devised the initial crude method of extracting the substance that would later be named insulin. Later, Collip refined the extraction process. Campbell and Fletcher oversaw the administration of the extract to 14-year-old Leonard Thompson. Macleod, as head of the University of Toronto's Department of Physiology, took a chance on Banting's idea and provided financial, logistical and intellectual support.
>
> (Hooey, 2000: 6)[2]

From this account one can immediately see the difficulty in identifying authorship. Regardless of whose hand actually penned the article, the question of origination or begetting is complicated. One man may have had an initial idea but the input of several others, in different capacities, was critical. Perhaps it is no wonder that the question caused legendary rows. Another, more controversial account concerns another Nobel Prize winning research team. Thirty years after the discovery of insulin, Watson and Crick published the famous paper in *Nature* reporting their work on the structure of DNA, for which they also subsequently received the Nobel Prize. However, some commentators argue that a significant amount of the credit should have gone to Rosalind Franklin. The claim is that a colleague of Franklin's, Maurice

Wilkins, showed Watson examples of Franklin's crystallographic portraits of DNA. Watson and Crick had been working on the problem of the structure of DNA and Franklin's X-ray picture enabled them very rapidly to solve the problem and publish their results. In their paper Watson and Crick acknowledge in a footnote that they 'have also been stimulated by knowledge of the general nature of the unpublished experimental results and ideas of Dr M H F Wilkins, Dr R E Franklin and their co-workers' (Watson and Crick, 1953: 737). If, as has been claimed, the breakthrough by Watson and Crick resulted from being shown Franklin's crystallographic portraits, the visual image providing the key trigger for their account, acknowledging that they had been 'stimulated by a knowledge of the general nature of the unpublished experimental results and ideas' of Franklin seems, shall we say, less than generous.[3]

The people who have the unenviable job of controlling the process of publication are the editors of scientific journals. The editors of medical journals have issued guidelines on authorship, which were revised in May 2000 and again in October 2005 (International Committee of Medical Journal Editors, 2005). Known as the Vancouver Guidelines these state in II.a that:

Authorship and contributorship credit should be based only on:

1   substantial contributions to conception and design, or acquisition of data, or analysis and interpretation of data;
2   drafting the article or revising it critically for important intellectual content; and
3   final approval of the version to be published.

Conditions 1, 2 and 3 must all be met. The authors of the International Council for Medical Journal Editors guidelines capture the sentiment behind their guidelines in a memorably pithy phrase: 'all persons designated as authors should qualify for authorship, and all those who qualify should be listed' (2005: 6). Acquisition of funding, the collection of data or general supervision of the research group, by themselves, do not justify authorship. This will be news to certain laboratory directors, who have argued that the very significant labour that is involved in gaining equipment, calibrating it, setting up protocols, winning research grants for materials and so on, thus qualifies them for authorship of ensuing publications.

Many journals now require that when a multi-authored manuscript is submitted each author must state his or her contribution and the days when a head of an academic department could expect to have his or her name on anything published by a member of staff or a researcher in the department, by a kind of *droit de seigneur*, are pretty much over.

Despite a very gradual shift aware from this practice, however, there still appear to be problems. Most people are well aware that much of the development of new drugs is funded and led by the pharmaceutical industry. The major drug companies invest huge amounts of money in their laboratories in the search for effective new compounds. When they have a promising candidate that is going to progress beyond Phase I trials and be given to human subjects suffering from the condition for which the drug is thought to be effective, the companies will find medical practitioners with whom they can collaborate. This is necessary because only through clinicians can they gain access to the population of sufferers for whom the drug may be used. One such clinician will usually be appointed as the principal investigator and, depending on the size of the study, others will be recruited as local investigators. When the trial is complete and favourable results have been obtained the information will be published in the relevant journals, probably with the principal investigator as first author.

Nevertheless, there is a widespread perception in academic circles that very often the articles are ghost-written by drug company staff, rather than by the actual investigators. Such practices may not breach the first of the three criteria in the Vancouver guidelines: we can assume that, while the trial will probably have been designed and managed by the drug company, the clinicians involved will have had significant input into the collection or acquisition of the data; and the company's staff will have conducted the analysis. However, condition 2 and possibly condition 3 are more problematic.

The World Association of Medical Editors (WAME) has recently published guidance on this area. They write:

> The integrity of the published record of scientific research depends not only on the validity of the science but also on honesty in authorship. Editors and readers need to be confident that authors have undertaken the work described and have ensured that the manuscript accurately reflects their work, irrespective of whether they took the lead in writing or sought assistance from a medical writer. The scientific record is distorted if the primary purpose of an article is to persuade readers in favor of a special interest, rather than to inform and educate, and this purpose is concealed.
>
> (WAME, 2005)

They advise editors in the following way:

> To prevent some instances of ghost authorship, editors should make clear in their journal's information for authors that medical writers can be legitimate contributors and that their roles and affiliations should be described in the manuscript. When editors detect ghost written manuscripts, their actions should involve both the submitting authors and commercial participants if they are involved. Several actions are possible:
>
> 1 publish a notice that a manuscript has been ghost written, along with the names of the responsible companies and the submitting author;

2   alert the authors' academic institutions, identifying the commercial companies;
3   provide specific names if contacted by the popular media or government organizations; and
4   share their experiences on the WAME Listserve and within other forums.

They argue that to these norms will not only deter the collusion of authors and commercial companies, but will greatly enhance the transparency of published scientific material and will also assist in the accountability of authors for the works which they (allegedly) publish.

Plagiarism

The idea of plagiarism, the copying of someone else's work and passing it off as one's own, sometimes seems to cause amusement. Tom Lehrer once wrote

Plagiarize,
Let no one else's work evade your eyes,
Remember why the good Lord made your eyes,
So don't shade your eyes,
But plagiarize, plagiarize, plagiarize . . .
Only be sure always to call it please, *'research'*.

(Lehrer, 1953)

His wit is only exceeded in accuracy by the Thompson (1957) quote 'To crib from one book is plagiarism, to crib from a dozen is research; to crib from any larger number will get you a doctorate of philosophy from one of the less exacting universities' (cited in Kitsburg, 2001: 226).

According to Eaton (2004) the problem of plagiarism is particularly rife among university students, with a recent survey suggesting that as many as one in four students admitted to having plagiarised the work of others when preparing assignments for their degrees. More publicly we have had the recent example of the British prime minister putting his name to a so-called dossier of evidence on the existence of weapons of mass destruction which turned out to have been largely copied from a doctoral thesis. Mr Blair (or, more likely, the unfortunate member of his staff who actually compiled the document) fell into one of the traps that await the unwary plagiarist, copying the text faithfully, complete with errors of punctuation.

But what is this thing called 'plagiarism'? Martin (1994) helpfully sets out some varieties:

1   Word-for-word plagiarism;
2   Plagiarism of secondary sources;
3   Plagiarism of the form of the source;

4   Plagiarism of ideas;
5   Plagiarism of authorship.

A brief discussion is necessary here for the distinctions can be subtle and it should be clear upon exposition that the varying types of plagiarism should exact differing levels of opprobrium.

Clearly, word-for-word plagiarism is the easiest form of plagiarism to detect. At one moment a teacher finds themselves wading through tortured grammar and prolix prose only to be confronted by a paragraph or two that Iris Murdoch or Ernest Hemingway would have been proud of – or rather, we should say, 'were proud of' – since they wrote it. There are now complex systems of detecting such fraud including the Joint Information Systems Committee (JISC) in the UK but simple cases may be detected through search engines simply by typing a phrase into the web.

Plagiarism of secondary sources is a more subtle matter. Where this is done inadvertently, as we believe it often is – and especially in the social sciences – it would not be proper to call it plagiarism. Clearly there is no intention to deceive.

It may be reasonable to think that plagiarism of secondary sources is perhaps more prevalent among brighter students, or even academics themselves. There are certain skills and understanding that must be brought to bear before one plagiarises secondary sources. This may be deceitful and it may not. Often doctoral students are in between – they are beginning to find their own authorial voice. They recognise that their work stands on the shoulders of others. If one is to err here, it is best that one does so, not so much on the side of caution, but of humility. Good supervisors will guide their students as to what is necessary and what is not regarding citations and references. Very often when one writes second or third drafts during the course of a thesis, one sees that points previously raised are commonplace in the literature and that the passage can be stated without a direct reference but can be paraphrased as a secondary reference. Sometimes the point will be so obvious, upon further research, that not even a secondary reference is necessary. It may well be the case that there are some interesting fault lines here according to the research discipline.

At this point it may be useful to rehearse a few further distinctions made by Martin, (1984: 183–4). The most obvious and provable plagiarism occurs when someone copies phrases or passages out of a published work without using quotation marks, without acknowledging the source, or both: word-for-word plagiarism. When some of the words are changed, but not enough, the result can be called paraphrasing plagiarism. This is considered more serious when the original source is not cited.

A more subtle plagiarism occurs when a person gives references to original sources, and perhaps quotes them, but never looks them up, having obtained both from a secondary source – which is not cited (Bensman, 1988, as cited in Martin, 1994: 456–7). This can be called plagiarism of secondary sources.

Often it can be detected through minor errors in punctuation or citation which are copied from the secondary source. More elusive yet is the use of the structure of the argument in a source without due acknowledgment of the source. This includes cases in which the plagiariser does look up the primary sources but does not acknowledge a systematic dependence on the citations in the secondary source. This can be called plagiarism of the form of a source. More general than this is plagiarism of ideas, in which an original thought from another is used but without any dependence on the words or form of the source. Finally there is the blunt case of putting one's name to someone else's work, which might be called plagiarism of authorship.

Martin asserts that much word-for-word plagiarism is inadvertent. With considerable compassion he writes:

> Undoubtedly, much of the word-for-word plagiarism by students is inadvertent. They simply do not know or understand proper acknow-ledgement practice. . . . Students are apprentices, and some of them learn the scholarly trade slowly.
>
> (Martin, 1994: 36)

Representatives of Georgetown University's Honor Council in the United States are both more cynical and – it seems reasonable to suggest – more realistic. To be sure some undergraduate students, often confronted with the need to reference ideas, find themselves uncertain as to how, and even why, such a need exists. For others the mistake is not one of naïveté but rather the vice of deceit. Georgetown University's Honor Council list the following 'would-be' innocent explanations:

1   They Said It So Much Better. Shouldn't I Use Their Words?
2   What is a Paraphrase, Anyway?
3   My Friends Get Stuff From the Internet.
4   I Don't Have Time to Do It Right.
5   A Citation is Not a Traffic Ticket.
6   What If My Roommate Helped Me?
7   In My Country/High School, Using Someone Else's Work is a Sign of Respect.

(http://gervaseprograms.georgetown.edu/hc/plagiarism.html,
accessed 6 January 2006)

Further explanation is scarcely necessary. Nevertheless, one can summarise as follows. Of course great scholars and scientists achieve status and recogni-tion properly by their research excellence. One should *appropriately* use their research and often their precise data or expressions. Paraphrasing is impo-rtant too, to show the examiner that students can sort the chaff from the wheat – use the best sources, discard poor research in favour of excellent, new from old, and so on. We all stand on the shoulders of those who go before us. But to paraphrase without acknowledging the source of the ideas is of course to pass someone's work off as one's own. Not only is this an instance of the vice of deceit, it is also unjust: the original source merits citation; they deserve it. And desert is a critical component of justice.[4]

In addition, they list three clear criteria that should be used to determine the need to reference. Appropriately they acknowledge (and so do we!) the original source to be that of Cornell University:

1   If you use someone else's ideas, you should cite the source.
2   If the way in which you are using the source is unclear, make it clear.
3   If you received specific help from someone in writing the paper, acknowledge it

(http://gervaseprograms.georgetown.edu/hc/index.html)

In the UK the JISC has led the development of plagiarism detection (http://www.submit.ac.uk/static_jisc/ac_uk_index.html) using a leading US plagiarism software company iParadigms, and offer advice and guidance to academics and students alike (http://www.jiscpas.ac.uk/). This allows comparisons between an alleged author's work and previously published material.

Plagiarism by students is widely acknowledged as a form of cheating, which may give the student an unfair advantage when it comes to the final degree classification and this is clearly a serious problem. In academic research, however, the unacknowledged copying of the work of others is an even more serious offence, essentially amounting to the theft of someone else's property. As Martin puts it: 'Among intellectuals, plagiarism is normally treated as a grievous sin' (1994: 36). Student essays do not appear on one's CV as publications and thus do not count towards such things as appointments to academic posts, or the awarding of chairs or research grants.

Zawadzki and Abbasi (1998) report the case of Dr Andrzej Jendryczko, who was working at the time of the publication of Zawadzki and Abbasi's article at the environmental engineering department at the Polytechnic Institute of Czestochowa and had previously worked at the Medical University of Silesia, where he had been Professor of Biochemistry. From a search of scientific databases it appeared that Jendryczko had published 125 papers in 13 years, but his accusers allege that at least 30 of these were plagiarised. In some cases he is alleged to have simply translated an English-language publication into Polish and then passed it off as his own work, while in others he apparently constructed new papers by taking sections of other published work and cutting and pasting them to make a new article.

Given the drive to maximise publications, authors who would not dream of passing off the work of another as their own may be guilty of what we might call auto-plagiarism, the recycling of passages from one of their own publications in another. It is not uncommon for researchers to publish several papers in different journals, drawing from the same piece of research. This can be quite legitimate, as one may publish a paper describing some particular problem of research methods and design (e.g. Wallace *et al.*, 2002a), and then a paper reporting the principal findings of the study (e.g. Wallace *et al.*, 2002b) and perhaps finally a further paper discussing a specific sub-element of the study (e.g. Jacklin *et al.*, 2003). The observant reader will spot the name of one of the authors of this book in all three of those papers, which cover quite separate aspects of the research and will be of interest to different readerships. However, it is also almost inevitable that in some passages these papers will bear striking resemblances to each other. It is a matter of subtle judgement, therefore, to know when the earlier papers should be acknowledged. Clearly editors prefer wholly new research data or theory but this notion is not universally acknowledged or followed.

Research fraud

One interesting example of alleged research fraud is *The Case of the Midwife Toad* (Koestler, 1974). This concerns the story of Paul Kammerer, a Viennese biologist, who committed suicide on 23 September 1926. Kammerer had never accepted Darwin's theory of evolution, preferring instead the account of Lamarck, of the inheritance of acquired characteristics. Koestler's book about Kammerer makes fascinating reading but, in brief, Kammerer devoted his experimental work to trying to prove Lamarck's theory. He worked particularly with amphibians, and the project that led to his suicide involved *Alytes Obstetricans*, the midwife toad. Most other toads mate in water, and the male toads have so-called nuptial pads, spiny areas on their forelimbs that allow them to grip the female's wet body. Midwife toads mate on dry land and have dry, rough skin, so these pads are not necessary and the males have none. Kammerer forced his captive-bred toads to mate in water, in the expectation that, as a result of their changed envrionment, they would acquire nuptial pads and that these would then be inherited by future generations, in keeping with Lamarckian theory. Kammerer claimed to have succeeded in this work, publishing papers and exhibiting specimens of midwife toads that showed the pads. However, when one of Kammerer's critics had the opportunity to examine one of the specimens he found no trace of the spiny pads and that the dark pigmented area where the pads would be appeared to have been created by injecting Indian ink into the skin of the toad. It is by no means certain that Kammerer faked this data himself, and Koestler's book goes into some detail about the claims and counter-claims, the possibility that an over-zealous laboratory assistant had produced the fakes and so on. Whatever the truth, Kammerer must have felt that his reputation was ruined and decided to take his own life.

Accounts of fraud in the biology laboratories of 1920s Austria may seem the stuff of television drama, but removed from (by some distance) twenty-first-century scientific research. Unfortunately this is not the case. In 1997, for example, the legal correspondent of the *British Medical Journal* (Dyer, 1997) reported the case of John Anderton, an Edinburgh renal consultant.

Dr Anderton, a former registrar and secretary of the Royal College of Physicians in Edinburgh, was struck off the medical register when he admitted falsifying data in a drug trial. He fabricated patients' consent forms and their data, creating fake echocardiograph and magnetic resonance imaging data for 17 patients. An extraordinary aspect of the story is that, according to the *British Medical Journal* report, he made no personal gain from his fraud and actually had to do more work to falsify the data than he would have if he had conducted the trial properly.

The year after the Anderton case, the BBC reported findings from the Committee on Publication Ethics suggesting at least 25 further examples of fraudulent research, including an example remarkably similar to the Kammerer case: a scientist reported that he had successfully transplanted black skin onto a white mouse, but on examination it was found that he had simply coloured the mouse skin with the modern equivalent of India ink, a black felt-tip pen. Dyer (2003) also reports the case of Goran Jamal, who falsified data in a drug trial conducted for a company which had promised him a share of any profits if the drug were successfully licensed and marketed. Pownall (1999) reports yet another review of research fraud in which the US Office of Research Integrity found that of 150 cases investigated, fraud was found in 76, mostly falsification or fabrication of data but also plagiarism.

Perhaps most spectacularly of all, the most recent case of research fraud, with global significance, is that of Hwang Woo-suk of Seoul University, South Korea. In 2004 he had claimed to have cloned stem cells – a medical breakthrough with inestimable implication for future health care (Woo-suk, 2004). After it was confirmed that donor eggs had been obtained from researchers engaged in the project, and that several co-authors had withdrawn their support for the research, several scientific bulletin boards queried the status of the research.[5] In December 2005, the news of his fabrication of data hit the headlines across the world. Having appeared in the highly prestigious journal *Science*, the article has now been retracted. Moreover, in letters and corrections to the journal in December 2005 it was noted that:

> Contrary to the statements in the second paragraph of text and first paragraph of the supporting online material, which indicated that there was no financial payment to oocyte and cumulus cell donors, some oocyte donors were financially compensated for their donation with a payment of approximately U.S. $1,400.

It appears that this spectacular fall from grace is the exception rather than the rule. Few will believe the principal investigator's early protestations that the deception had been carried out by research assistants on him:

> We believe they completely deceived [us] with their research results. Relying on the role and responsibility of Mizmedi hospital, we trusted their reports 100%.

Or succumb to his comments on the pressure of research:

> We were crazy, crazy about work, [he said] I was blinded. All I could see
> was whether I could make Korea stand in the centre of the world
> through this research.
>
> (http://www.guardian.co.uk/korea/article/0,,1684859,00.html,
> accessed 2 February 2006)

Moreover, there will be fewer still who will feel the slightest sympathy for
him. They will, however, be moved more by thought of the communities of
sufferers for whom genuine genetic-technological breakthroughs are seen as a
last hope.

Whistleblowing and sanctions on offenders[6]

In the leading academic weekly newspaper in the UK, the *Times Higher Education Supplement*, there has appeared over the last few years a specific column
entitled 'Whistleblower'. In its columns have been various calumnies against
integrity in academic life. But what, specifically, is meant by whistleblowing?
Its derivation is contested. Geoffrey Hunt asserts that it probably owes its
genesis to referees or umpires, who draw attention to a foul in a game by blowing a whistle. Conversely, it has been claimed, 'Whistleblowing has been derived from the act of British constables after the commission of a crime to warn
the public of any danger and to alert other law enforcement officers in the
area' (see http://exodus.broward.cc.fl.us/pathfinders/whistleblowing.htm).

Given that the origins of the term are uncertain it should be no surprise
that more than one theory of whistleblowing exists. What can generally, and
incontestably, be said is that whistleblowing entails the revealing of information to prevent or to bring about the cessation of a significant wrong within
an organisation, by a person within that organisation.

Bok characterises the general aim of whistleblowing thus: the alarm of the
whistleblower is intended to disrupt the status quo: to pierce the background
noise, perhaps the false harmony or the imposed silence of 'affairs as usual'
(1988: 332). She then sets out three morally salient features of whistleblowing: dissent, breach of loyalty and accusation of wrongdoing. If we agree
roughly upon these features, we must recognise the salience[7] of two issues:
the right of innocents (such as co-authors or research students or colleagues)
not to be harmed or exploited and the conflict raised herein by the breach
of loyalty to the university or the department/faculty/school (though there
are many more complicating factors, as I have noted). The whistleblower
must consider how these factors enter into justifications of their act of
whistleblowing.

Davis (1996: 6–7) argues that the received or standard theory[8] recognises
that an act of whistleblowing is *prima facie* an act of disloyalty that may be
justified when three conditions apply.

1   The organization to which the would-be whistleblower belongs, through its product or policy, [does] serious harm to the public. . . .
2   The would-be whistleblower has identified the threat of harm, reported it to her immediate superior, making clear both the threat itself and the objection to it, and concluded that the superior will do nothing effective; and
3   The would-be whistleblower has exhausted other internal procedures within the organization . . . or at least made use of as many internal procedures as the danger to others and her own safety make reasonable.

If conditions 1–3 are satisfied, whistleblowing is morally justifiable, according to what Michael Davis calls the 'standard theory'. We should, however, note his emphasis on the duties or obligations of the would-be whistleblower to exhaust internal mechanisms of the organisation first. This is an inherently conservative position. The very mechanisms and ethos of the institution may well display sexist, racist or other unethical dimensions which might lead a reasonable person to conclude that the internal mechanisms (or lack of them) are themselves part of the problem.

But, arguably, a more serious issue is Davis's position that whistleblowing is obligatory if the further conditions prevail:

4   The would-be whistleblower has (or has accessible) evidence that would convince a reasonable, impartial observer that her view of the threat is correct; and
5   The would-be whistleblower has good reason to believe that revealing the threat will (probably) prevent the harm at reasonable cost (all things considered).

First, let us note here the deontological approach: framing a universalisable obligation in terms of principles. We have argued in Chapter 2 that it is the matrix of factors particular to a case that help us to make casuistic judgements about research ethics: this will include the moral salience of our felt emotions and ethical judgements about right character and conduct.

How would these considerations alter our attitude to criterion 4? For instance, what sense can be made of the idea of an 'impartial observer'? As we have noted, the idea of a view from nowhere is a non-starter; a throwback to a naïve view of science and a rationalist conception of ethics. Emotions and their corresponding judgements can only arise in the light of particular situations. Indeed, the very idea of moral perception or moral salience presupposes a situated agent, one in a position to see the conflict. The fifth criterion is even more problematic. What sense are we to make of the idea of an obligation (a moral duty upon the researcher) to blow a whistle upon the basis of a consequentialist calculation of costs and benefits? It is ordinarily thought that duties themselves are precisely a means to secure minimal moral standards that prevent people being treated disrespectfully or harmed unreasonably. The idea that an obligation only arises when the benefits out-weigh the costs runs counter to the very idea of obligation. If this is not so, why would one not simply be a utilitarian: ascertain the facts of pleasures and pains, utility and disutility and then blow the whistle or not?

Now if all this seems less than satisfactory, it should be underlined that Davis argues for a revised version of the standard theory. The details of Davis's critique need not detain us here (notwithstanding its prominence within the professional ethics literature) except for the specific moral rele-vance he places upon the intra-organisational character of the whistleblower and her acts. It is on the basis of this that he renames the theory as the 'complicity theory': the obligation to blow the whistle derives from the complicity of the whistleblower rather than the mere ability or inclination to prevent harm. Davis claims that the agent in such cases enters the situation voluntarily. No-one has coerced them to work in this or that institution. It seems, however, that he is wrenching the right cause in the wrong way. He recognises the fact that voluntariness is not a necessary condition for justify-ing whistleblowing but argues that 'involuntary participants will not have the same obligation of loyalty as the typical whistleblower; hence any theory justifying their "going public" will have a somewhat different structure than the theory developed here' (1996: 18) He also makes much of the insider–outsider status of the would-be whistleblower. This distinction is commonly labelled internal and external whistleblowing.

Nevertheless, what researchers may well feel most strongly about in their quandaries as to whether to blow the whistle or not, may not be a deep felt sense of loyalty to their acadmic institutions *simpliciter* but the attention to the harm that will be caused to innocent others. In any event there needs to be some conception of a degree of detachment; working within the organisa-tion should not in itself be taken to imply complicity. Now in some cases there may well be some complicity on behalf of the person who is consider-ing blowing the whistle, but this can often be thought of as bad moral luck in cases where the individual merely finds themselves implicated in the wrongdoing, and not morally responsible for it.

Furthermore, there are other self-regarding reasons that will weigh with researchers here, and they should not be dismissed lightly. In attempting to make our judgement as to whether we are obliged to blow the whistle, we are forced seriously to ask what constitutes 'a reasonable cost' and who is to be included in the counting that delivers the calculation? Many whistleblowers themselves fare pretty badly. To start with, whistleblowing is at odds with three significantly important institutional considerations: the need for con-formity with organisational cultures;[9] the requirement of adherence to pro-fessional standards (including collegiality); and the dynamics of institutional loyalty (Gadlin, 1998). Whistleblowers often end up paying a very heavy price.[10] Joan Sieber notes the chilling advice of one whistleblower from the Environmental Protection Agency, the fruit of bitter experience:

Don't make the mistake of thinking that someone in authority, if he only knew what was going on, would straighten the whole thing out. If you have God, the law, the press, and the facts on your side, you have a fifty-fifty chance of defeating the bureaucracy.

(Sieber, 1988: 25)[11]

A final related point made frequently in the literature is that of the need for examination of one's motives. Whistleblowers ought not to be seen to profit from their blowing of the whistle; they should do it for entirely moral reasons, or so it is generally thought (James, 1988). This takes us back to the way that those with feminist and other overt political commitments, more so than those without, will weigh certain conduct more heavily. The self-same facts that may be seen as exploitative by one might appear merely inappropriate to another. If the whistleblower is seen to be advancing their cause, having an axe to grind, her chances of arousing the relevant community, of shouting 'foul' loud and clear in a way that compels professional support, will greatly diminish. Often less overt leakage is the minimal-damage route through to a clear conscience (Eraut, 1984). Either way, a careful examination of their motives, and their perception of the facts, will be critical if the whistleblowing is to succeed and whistleblowers are to be sure that they have done the right thing for the right reason at the right time.

Dealing with research misconduct in relation to individuals is not something that has reached an advance state. Calls for a national response have been made in the UK since at least 1998 (Rennie, 1998; Smith, 1998).[12]

One clear problem is that once researchers have had the whistle blown on them, and the fraud publicly reported, whose job is it to follow up on all previously published reports or papers? Take the example of the Canadian nutritionist Chandra, who recently had his article retracted from *Nutrition* (White, 2004). Smith (2005) gives an account of how he, as editor of the *British Medical Journal* had rejected the paper on the advice of reviewers, one of whom had claimed it bore all the hallmarks of an entirely invented paper. When Chandra's employers, the Memorial University of Newfoundland, were asked to follow up they found no serious problem. When the editor of *Nutrition* communicated eight reasons why the article should be retracted, the author did not respond, nor did he respond to requests for raw data. Later that year he resigned.

The prospect for the future is that of an approach which will continue typically to be piecemeal. This will be because of the difficulties of different international legal frameworks, different disciplinary traditions of research and research governance. It may also be because of the infrequency with which it occurs. It may just as well be because it is the kind of news that universities, like any other institutions, want to keep private. Public retractions, such as those in the Korean stem cell research case, can only serve as a powerful disincentive to research fraudsters at such a powerful international level. What happens below this is, as they say, likely to be 'below the radar'.

Nevertheless, the Committee on Publication Ethics advises every editor, *inter alia*, to have procedures in place to support the reporting of research misconduct, and so too should every university, IRB or REC.

Parafraud?

Having discussed issues of plagiarism and fraud in general terms it is worth noting the shape they take in summary form and specifying further some particularly prevalent examples. Hillman (1998) draws attention to practices that he calls 'parafraud', practices that include:

- authors not publishing results that do not support their hypotheses;
- authors not doing crucial control experiments;
- authors claiming authorship of papers towards which they have not made any contribution;
- authors leaving out some results of experiments arbitrarily;
- referees recommending rejection of papers for publication without specifying reasons and relevant references, or rejecting work that may yield results throwing into doubt the value of their own work;
- referees recommending that grants not be given to fund research by competitors;
- authors misquoting other authors deliberately or accidentally;
- referees not reading manuscripts or submissions for grants with sufficient attention to assess them seriously;
- authors not answering questions at meetings or in correspondence;
- authors ignoring findings inimical to, or preceding, their own;
- authors being unwilling to discuss their own published research.

The worrying thing is that Hillman claims of these practices 'that most of them are regarded as acceptable by the academic community'. This may well be to generalise inappropriately though. As we have said throughout this book, there is a particular need to be sensitive to the subtle nuances of each discipline's own research tradition.

Hillman's concerns are echoed by Al-Marzouki *et al.* (2005). These authors conducted a Delphi study in which their expert panel identified 60 forms of scientific misconduct which they agreed were likely or very likely to distort the results of a clinical trial. Of these, the panel identified 13 forms of misconduct that were both likely to distort results and were likely or very likely to occur:

- Over-interpretation of significant findings in small trials
- Selective reporting based on p-values
- Selective reporting of outcomes in the abstract
- Subgroup analyses done without interaction tests
- Negative or detrimental studies not published

- Putting undue stress on results from subgroup analysis
- Inappropriate subgroup analyses
- Selective reporting of (i) subgroups (ii) outcomes (iii) time points
- Selective reporting of positive results or omission of adverse events data
- Failure to report results or long delay in reporting
- Post-hoc analysis not admitted
- Giving incomplete information about analyses with non-significant results
- Analysis conducted by the sponsor of the trial.

The authors note that:

> Although there has been considerable attention in the scientific literature on the problems of data fabrication and data falsification these were absent from our list of the most important forms of misconduct because there was majority agreement that these problems were very unlikely to occur.
>
> (Al-Marzouki *et al.*, 2005: 7)

As we have seen, this is a view not entirely supported by the literature.

Conclusion: reconceptualising research as a practice, and a sketch of a more ethical research culture

Somewhat counter-intuitively, though entirely in keeping with his consequentalist utilitarian perspective, Bentham once wrote that:

> Falsehood, taken by itself, consider it as not being accompanied by any other material circumstances, nor therefore productive of any material effects, can never, upon the principal of utility, constitute any offence at all.

To be fair he also suggests:

> Combined with other circumstances, there is scarce any sort of pernicious effect which it may not be instrumental in producing.
>
> (cited in Bok, 1978b: 47)

The view that falsehood is acceptable so long as it does not produce bad consequences cannot find a foothold in research ethics, for the purpose of research is to aim at the truth (or some version thereof).

We suggested at the beginning of this chapter that the pressures on academics and scientists are such that the temptation to commit fraud in research is severe. Skinner (1998) sums this up in a letter to the *British Medical Journal* in which he argues that a key problem in the UK is that research output (i.e. publications) is used as a yardstick of performance when making appointments in the National Health Service, a yardstick that outweighs all others. The same is true for universities and no doubt for other institutions: in the UK it is a particular problem in the system of the assessment of the quality of research in a department, on which substantial sums of money and even the future survival of the department may depend. As Skinner says:

> Academic departments retain funding, award tenure, and make appointments largely on the basis of research published, albeit with lip service being paid to an assessment of quality. Excellence in teaching seems an irrelevance. Is it any wonder that people embellish or even invent results?
>
> (Skinner, 1998: x)

The relationship between practices and institutions is a complex one, as MacIntyre (1984) reminds us. Practices require institutions in which to take place, but they have very different goals and objectives and quite different agendas. For MacIntyre, practices are characterised by, among other things, the necessity of the moral virtues and the status of the goods with which the practice may be associated. The virtues MacIntyre sees as core to a practice are those of honesty, courage and justice. The goods associated with a practice he divides into those internal to the practice and those external to it. Internal goods would be those things that can only be experienced through engagement with the practice: the satisfaction of achievement of the ends to which the practice is directed, the striving after excellence on the part of the practitioner and so on. For a researcher these would include the creation of new knowledge in the researcher's chosen field and, possibly, the translation of that knowledge into some benefit to society. So, for the sports scientist perhaps, there would be gratification from seeing a reduction in the incidence of injuries that may be the result of innovative work on training techniques, while the physician will derive satisfaction from the increased effectiveness of a new treatment for some medical complaint.

Interestingly, however, this instrumental value of research may not be a necessary condition for the acquisition of internal goods: for many, the acquisition of knowledge has intrinsic value, regardless of whether there is any eventual application or not. Researchers would also, we presume, derive internal goods from the satisfaction that comes from improving skills, techniques and methods, both at the personal level of individual competence and from the development of new techniques that will help to advance research methodology across the field.

The virtues have a critical part to play because, for MacIntyre, the goods internal to the practice cannot be enjoyed unless the practitioner exhibits the moral virtues, or courage, honesty and justice among others. The reasoning, put simply, is that the satisfaction we gain from succeeding at something difficult melts away if we cheat. We have to have the courage to face up to the difficulties inherent in what we attempt, we have to have the honesty to acknowledge our failures and our shortcomings, and we have to be just in our acknowledgement of the contributions of others. Any pleasure experienced by Jendryczko from his plagiarised publications must have come from the knowledge that he had successfully hoodwinked the editors and the scientific community: it cannot have come from any sense of excellence in scholarship because he knew the work was not his.

As already mentioned, there are real problems about the relationship between the practice of research and the institutions within which research is conducted. There are clear potential conflicts between the need of the institution for example to maximise income and, if income is dependent, directly or indirectly, on publication records, then there will be powerful but possibly perverse incentives on staff to get publications into prestigious journals by fair means or foul. The trouble is that what may start by being seen as totally unacceptable may become routine and unremarkable.

7 Ethics in qualitative research

The emergence of qualitative research

It is common knowledge that qualitative research uses methods that are different from those employed in quantitative studies. Some studies combine both of course and so we make a cautionary note at the beginning of the chapter that it is somewhat artificial to set out these two as competitors of some kind. It is true, however, that qualitative research may present a set of ethical challenges because of the closer relations between the researcher and researched. Given that methods impinge on ethical issues, it follows that there may be some differences in the ethical problems faced by the two sets of researchers.

There is evidence that researchers in the health sphere find the Research Ethics Committee (REC) approval process frustrating and qualitative research proposals are perceived to be particularly problematic (Hannigan and Allen, 2003). Not only do qualitative researchers face ethical problems that may be different to those inherent in quantitative work (Peled and Leichentritt, 2002), but also it has been contended that qualitative researchers may be treated unfairly by RECs and Institutional Research Boards (IRBs) (Ramcharan and Cutcliffe, 2001). Most ethics boards/committees are more familiar with quantitative methodologies, which could lead to inequitable treatment for qualitative researchers. This is particularly the case in sports and exercise science, where qualitative research is still a relatively new form of inquiry.

Nevertheless, despite initial resistance from traditional exercise and sports sciences practitioners, the role of qualitative research within the discipline is being increasingly accepted and valued; it is also gaining credibility (Biddle *et al.*, 2001; Allen-Collinson, 2005). Alternative methods, such as case studies, observational studies, ethnographies, action research and personal narrative histories, are being used with increasing frequency in areas such as the sociologies of health and sports, exercise and sports psychology, and sports management studies.

Even though the amount of qualitative research in exercise, health and sports sciences is increasing, the ubiquity of quantitative research in such research means that RECs are dominated by people versed in a positivist research methodology. A further problem faced by qualitative researchers when submitting their proposals for IRB/REC approval is that committee members may not be familiar with the sheer diversity of qualitative methods available to researchers.

In this chapter, we introduce and discuss some of the ethical issues raised by the use of different research approaches, as qualitative methodologies in some cases pose a different set of problems. We debate the applicability of the commonly applied biomedical ethics model for qualitative research, and take the perspective that judgements cannot simply be applied from an ideal-observer perspective which is attributable to the outdated positivistic philosophy of science.

Historical and conceptual context

The abuses perpetrated in invasive biomedical experiments, among other research, have already been documented in Chapter 1. As we saw in Chapter 3, the major response from research communities to these abuses was the formulation of the professional and international codes such as the Nuremberg Code, the Declaration of Helsinki and the many variations of IRB/REC approval processes in current operation.

The ethics review process initiated in response to research malpractice is founded on the basic principles of beneficence, non-maleficence (not harming research participants), justice and autonomy, as discussed in Chapter 2. Collectively, these principles aim to protect people from harm, to treat people equitably and to empower potential and actual participants. As we saw, these very general principles are often mixed, in theoretically unsatisfactory ways, with other appeals to utility and virtue, as well as with forms of reasoning that rely on precedent as much as principle.

Perhaps the dominant principle in research ethics is respect for autonomy, and it is this principle which enshrines an individual's right to self-determination and is practised through the insistence on obtaining first-person, written, informed consent, as discussed in Chapter 4. Issues such as anonymity, coercion and the right to withdraw from a project without sanction, are underpinned by the commonly accepted ethical principles mentioned above.

It is worth noting that an individual's right to self-determination may at times be at odds with a communitarian model of research ethics, which extols beneficence (rather than merely non-maleficence), and may stress the importance of group rather than individual rights. Such a communitarian model may at times be more appropriate for qualitative work, particularly in ethnographic work or action research. IRBs/RECs at present are probably not adequately sensitised to alternative models of research ethics such as this.

The methods sections of research proposals presented to IRBs/RECs dealing with health research, and to ethics committees in exercise and sports sciences, are traditionally expected to provide evidence of control of independent and extraneous variables, to describe relatively inflexible procedures (for good reasons of validity and reliability, it must be noted), and to present predetermined methods of analysis. As such, the majority of research proposal submissions in exercise and sports sciences tend to follow the tradition of the biomedical model. However, the positivistic perspective as enshrined in the biomedical model and guidelines of IRBs/RECs may be too inflexible for qualitative studies.

From biomedical to humanistic research in exercise, health and sports sciences

In the humanistic model of social research, Brewer suggests that:

> Stress is also laid on the analysis of people's meanings from their own standpoint: the feelings, perceptions, emotions, thoughts, moods, ideas, beliefs, and interpretative processes of members of society as they themselves understand and articulate them.
>
> (Brewer, 2000: 6)

In contrast, experimental biomedical research (including traditional models of exercise, health and sports science research), involves making every effort to exclude these 'feelings, perceptions, emotions, thoughts, moods, ideas and beliefs' through prospective design, random allocation, double blinding, placebos and statistical plans. In short, extraneous and confounding variables are eliminated or controlled.

One of the key aspects of much qualitative work is an inductive approach and emergent design of studies (including the methods of sampling and the actual direction of the study). Also, qualitative researchers present their findings in a variety of ways, which differ markedly from the presentation of quantitative investigators. Extreme examples might include ethnodrama, and poetic representations (Sparkes, 2002; Rapport, 2004; Rapport *et al.*, 2005). A different perspective on ethics, one that suggests a more flexible approach and appreciation of ongoing decision processes, may be more applicable for the challenges facing qualitative researchers.

The idea of 'a flexible approach' may be anathema to ethics committee members steeped in the biomedical research and research ethics traditions. The exclusion of subjectivity is traditionally seen as central to the conduct of 'science', with generalisability being of critical importance. Qualitative researchers do not revere validity and reliability, valuing the somewhat analogous concepts of authenticity and trustworthiness instead (Sparkes, 1998; Allen-Collinson, 2005). For them, analysing thick, rich descriptions that may assist understanding in other contexts, is as important as any positivistically derived notion of generalisable data, and as important as the ability to generate other health related benefits for humanity (such as a new treatment procedure or drug).

Qualitative research and RECs/IRBs

What is the remit of ethics committees in general? Most fundamentally, they serve to evaluate the ethical acceptability of proposed research projects. As we saw in Chapter 3, these committees are of crucial importance in regulating research and preventing abuses, since investigators should not be the sole judges of whether their research conforms with generally accepted ethical codes and practices.

In addition to considering ethical issues, the role of committees has expanded in many cases to include a broad range of design issues, and to ensure relevant research of good quality. It is this shift from a narrow ethics evaluation to a broader methodological scrutiny that may present difficulties for qualitative research. This is particularly the case if a committee is dominated by people immersed in positivist paradigms.

Qualitative research has different methods, and often poses different problems to quantitative work. Cultural factors, emotional involvement, benefits to participants, and issues such as covert observations, power relationships between researchers and participants, and public versus private behaviour, while often present in quantitative research, may require greater consideration in qualitative projects.

Even so, it could be argued that the principles of non-maleficence, justice and autonomy apply equally to quantitative and qualitative research. As researchers, we ought to be beneficent (if we can, and at the least we should practise non-maleficence), and we ought to be just, when conducting our research. Similarly, we ought to respect an individual or group's right to self-determination where it is relevant in the context of a particular research project. With regard to the latter idea, then, it follows that blind adherence to informed consent is neither necessary nor desirable.

Unqualified acceptance or prescription of the autonomy-above-all model disqualifies, by definition, covert research and deceptive research. Indeed, informed consent and deception are mutually exclusive concepts. This is not, of course, to suggest that the principle of autonomy does not apply to qualitative work, nor that consent should be blithely overridden by qualitative researchers. Rather it is that the consent process *may* justifiably be overridden in certain instances. Some qualitative researchers probably agree that covert or deceptive work may be justified in some cases, but there is ongoing debate in this area. Indeed, the idea has a particularly troubled history (Homan, 2002, 2005). On a point of fairness it should also be noted that covert work and deception are sometimes utilised in quantitative work, such as in the single-blind placebo in drug trials.

The lack of agreement over the ethics of covert work is captured by the divergent reactions to Humphreys' (1970) 'classic' study on homosexuals noted in Chapter 1. He acted as a 'watch queen' at public toilets, thus befriending the men. Later, he traced them from their car licence plates, and ultimately questioned them in their homes under the guise of a different project. The work provided important information on stereotypes of homosexual men, but questions were raised as to the ethics of the project. Punch (1998) notes that, on the one hand, he received a prestigious award for his work, whereas, on the other, efforts were made to revoke his PhD.

Such examples serve to illustrate the quagmire of dilemmas facing ethics committees. These committees are often guided by the codes of ethics of professional organisations. As we have seen, sometimes it is simply unclear, however, which professional code or norm is appropriate to apply. This is in itself a potential problem, as almost all codes have a strong deontological basis.

Codes of ethics published by recognised associations, such as the British Psychological Society (BPS) and the British Sociological Association (BSA) provide general guidelines on the obligations of researchers on confidentiality, informed consent and use of deception. However, such codes are either too specific (consider the British Association of Sports and Exercise Sciences [BASES] disavowal of all deceptive research discussed in Chapter 4) or too general (for example 'respect the rights of research participants' – thus giving inadequate guidance to those unfamiliar with ethical issues). In the American College of Sports Medicine (ACSM) and BASES, there is very little overt (in the form of ethical codification) recognition of the ethical issues that affect qualitative work. This may be because organisations simply do not feel that qualitative work requires specific guidelines. In the UK the Economic and Social Research Council (ESRC) have just produced their research ethics framework, which is a substantial and valuable contribution to the more general debate (ESRC, 2006).

Further, there is little evidence of discussion of ethical considerations in the vast majority of published qualitative research reports within exercise and sports sciences. This is not a criticism of social scientific research but more likely a failure of the dominant research traditions in exercise and sports sciences to engage with mainstream social science *per se*. Health-related research fares better. In a review of qualitative studies in social work, Peled and Leichentritt (2002) concluded that the lack of overt discussion on ethical considerations in published papers implies that the responsibility for 'proper ethical conduct' lies within the individual researchers. There are inherent dangers with such a reliance on individual researchers, who have a vested interest in the research. Self-interest, ego and career demands mean that we are almost never the best judges of our own work. Independent review, while not sufficient, is necessary. Nevertheless, it may be that the relative youthfulness of qualitative traditions in exercise and sports sciences means that it is being disadvantaged by ethics committees, with these committees being strongly influenced by the practices of biomedical ethics.

There is certainly room for further critical professional discussion and debate about ethical considerations in qualitative work within exercise, health and sports sciences. Such debates might helpfully focus – though not slavishly – on the key principles outlined in Chapter 2, including not doing harm (non-maleficence), justice, autonomy (where relevant and appropriate), research-related benefits for participants and for others (beneficence), and researchers' technical competence. Recurring themes for ethical issues in relation to qualitative research in exercise health and sports include the role of the researcher; the desirability and necessity of informed consent; deception; covert research; the researcher's responsibility to informants, sponsors and colleagues; risks versus benefits; reciprocity and intervention; issues of relationships and 'leaving the field'; how participants are represented in reports; and how to deal with unforeseen ethical issues that emerge during and after the research.

Qualitative methods and issues

One of the potential pitfalls for qualitative research subjected to a quantitatively orientated tradition of ethics review is that the research design is often emergent in the research process. The inherent open-endedness of inductive approaches (for example, much ethnography, or research that uses snowballing techniques of gaining access and gathering data) means that developing research procedures is an ongoing process (Sugden, 2005). The nature of the problem to be investigated is fluid, incompletely determined at the beginning of the study, and subject to change as the study progresses. So, inherent within these research processes is the element that the design cannot be exhaustively described in advance for ethical review, but rather emerges over time. This is in sharp contrast to experimental research, which requires, by its very nature, detailed planning and control. In qualitative research, however, it is often neither possible nor desirable to provide ethics committees with concrete numbers of participants in advance of the study (nor an exhaustive list of the specific questions that will be asked).

In qualitative research, the nature of the procedures means that questions or lines of questioning may change according to the preliminary responses received. Indeed, the very focus of the project may change, with a new fundamental direction being pursued. For example, in a project investigating power relationships among sports coaches and young children, the initial focus might be on the coach–athlete relationship. It is conceivable though, that during the conduct of the research, it becomes apparent that the real determinant of the power situation is a notion of power being transferred from parents to the coach, and consequently exercised by the latter. Thus it might emerge that there are multiple sources of power, and the emphasis may switch to examining the alternatives, rather than solely focusing on the original supposition. So, at any stage of a qualitative project, the information received and concurrently evaluated can influence either or both the immediate procedures and the ultimate direction of the project. This is in contrast to more traditional areas of study in exercise, health and sports sciences.

For example, in a physiological study investigating time to exhaustion during energy drink and placebo conditions, the physiological risks are well established and risk can be managed through careful monitoring and appropriate emergency medical provision. If the subject has provided voluntary consent and has adequately comprehended the relevant information, the project is likely to be deemed ethically acceptable.

A qualitative project may be different, however, in that the problems are perhaps more difficult to foresee. This provides a challenge for qualitative researchers. For example, in examining group cohesion in sports teams, Fishwick (1983) found that a particular clique's fondness for illegal drugs was a major source of discord and affected team morale. This led to a series of unanticipated ethical issues concerning informant confidentiality, trust and decisions about what to include in the final report. Such unforeseen circumstances are not limited to the extended fieldwork of ethnographic research. Similarly, types of issues can also be revealed during in-depth interviewing. For example, an investigator wants to examine the influence of media images on perceptions of body image. During an interview it becomes clear that a participant suffers from a serious eating disorder. The researcher is not trained to deal with this. What ought s/he to do?

There is of course an answer to this moral issue, but this chapter is not the place to explore it.[1] Rather, the example serves to illustrate the differences in planning and procedure that could be experienced by quantitative and qualitative researchers. Researchers should plan adequately, and ethics committees should recognise that different approaches present different solutions and problems. One ethics process model will not, in cases such as these, cater adequately for all research proposals. Generally speaking, if procedures and ethical issues are adequately considered and catered for in advance, then the project is more likely to be deemed ethically acceptable. For example, in his participant observation work on soccer hooligans, it is likely that Giulianotti (1995) considered in advance his guidelines for action if he himself were faced with actual involvement in physical violence. Sugden (1995, 2002) goes further and suggests that one must expect such difficulties from time to time in certain lines of ethnographic research. A rarer example of a more detailed and considered approach to guidelines of personal responsibility is given by Brackenridge (2001). In her account of how she managed the interview process (which focused on sexual exploitation of athletes) she explicitly mentions oral consent procedures, confidentiality agreements, storage of data, participant input, follow-up counselling arrangements, and her stance of non-involvement in reporting on behalf of a participant.

We are not arguing here that qualitative researchers should be singled out in terms of attempting to predict potential issues in their research, as such forethought is of course also needed for quantitative studies. It does not follow that ethical problems should be approached differently for different types of research. Whatever relativists would have us believe, and as we have tried to illustrate thus far, there are ethical considerations that ought to be considered when planning and evaluating any research project. We have attempted to illustrate how very general ethical considerations may be over-ridden in certain circumstances yet this does not mean that non-maleficence, justice and autonomy can be ignored. Particularly for qualitative research, beneficence where possible (in terms of the immediate participants), should also be considered here.

Specific issues that all researchers need to consider are the nature of confi-dentiality agreements, anonymity, privacy, risks and benefits (physical, social, psychological), consent and deception, covert observation, cultural and/or gender factors, using vulnerable populations, coercion and sanction in the participation process, the researcher's response to harmful/stressful situ-ations (for both participant and researcher), the desirability and nature of debriefing, and how emerging and ongoing ethical issues will be dealt with.

Consent requirements and guidelines

The principle of autonomy, embracing an individual's right to self-determination, underpins the notion of informed consent as we saw in Chapter 4. Informed consent implies that a participant freely agrees to par-ticipate (without coercion or threat of sanction being applied), and that the relevant consequences of such an agreement are understood by him/her. In studies where the notion of informed consent is considered appropriate, it is preferable that it is obtained in written form, and that it is given by the person concerned (first-person consent). This is intended to protect both the investigator and the research participant.

Many IRBs/RECs, in applying the biomedical ethics model, will insist on written, first-person informed consent being obtained. This may not always be appropriate, however, even in quantitative studies. For example, if researchers wish to investigate energy expenditure among illiterate isiZulu-speaking cane-cutters in Africa (perhaps with the laudable aim of improving working conditions), they would find that written first-person informed con-sent is inappropriate (see Chapter 9 for a full consideration of such issues). The first and most obvious problem is illiteracy. The second issue is that, generally speaking, a community such as the research population described above subscribes to a notion of community-based rights and decision-making, rather than the essentially Western notion of individualism. In this case, individually witnessed oral consent may be appropriate, if obtained in conjunction with permission from, for example, a tribal elder. It is worth noting that such consent needs to be contemporaneously recorded in writing, with this recording being witnessed if possible.

The applicability of informed consent may vary according to the charac-teristics of the participants. When young children are involved, parental (proxy) consent plus the child's assent (agreement) is necessary. For older children, proxy consent and a modified (comprehensible)[2] consent form should be employed. I would contend that, when using children as participants, active consent procedures should be applied, as opposed to passive consent. Vulnerable populations such as prisoners or people with learning disabilities (for example), need special considerations to be applied (such as paying particular attention to comprehensibility; being aware of the potential for coercion; and so on).

A marked difference between consent requirements for qualitative and quantitative research relates to those of whom consent is asked and whether consent is needed at more than one point in time. We referred to this in Chapter 4 as the 'process' of informed consent. When using open-ended interviewing, questions often go down avenues not anticipated by the researcher or the participant. An example of research of this nature would be Sparkes' (1996; Sparkes and Smith, 2003) work on life history and narratives of self. While work such as this may seem to be 'unplanned' to quantitative researchers, it is of course an integral part of the exploratory, emergent nature of some qualitative work. In cases such as this, or if using covert observation, behaviours may take unexpected directions and the distinction between public and private behaviour may become very blurred, such as in Whyte's (1943) classic *Street Corner Society* study. The data obtained may be extremely valuable, but does the original consent agreement cover unsolicited and unanticipated disclosures? Will such unexpected directions increase the likelihood of participants making further unwanted disclosures? Also, qualitative researchers need to consider whether or not their consent agreement includes issues relating to participant involvement in the transcription and reporting process. Will participants have the opportunity to check transcripts, and what will be their rights in terms of deleting (perhaps sensitive) information?

The possibilities outlined in the preceding paragraph suggest that in qualitative studies, such as ethnographic work, action research and narrative life history (involving a series of interviews), informed consent is not a single event. Rather, obtaining informed consent is an ongoing process in which the researcher has to be sensitive to participants' reactions during data collection, and be prepared to renegotiate consent every now and then (see Chapter 4). IRBs/RECs need to be aware that, in qualitative work, the nature and direction of a project can change, thus changing the nature of the consent requirements. Both ethics committees and researchers must identify mechanisms whereby such changes can be communicated and facilitated. Given the relative youth of qualitative inquiry in exercise, health and sports sciences, we suggest that it might be prudent for researchers themselves to lead the way by explicitly including ethics review and monitoring procedures in their research proposals to committees.

Deceptive research

Obtaining informed consent in qualitative research sometimes poses problems. Many of the classic sports ethnographies, such as Fine's (1987) study of little league baseball, Klein's (1993) study of male bodybuilders and Crossett's (1995) study of women's professional golf, would not have been conducted if written consent was required of all the participants within these sports subcultures. Deception and informed consent are, as previously mentioned, mutually exclusive concepts. So, by definition, if an ethics committee insists absolutely on consent, it cannot logically approve studies involving deception. Ethics committees are generally wary of approving studies that require deception, and researchers are advised to present strong justifications if they intend proposing such methods. It may thus be up to researchers to convince a committee that deception in a study can be justified.

So, along with current trends in IRB/REC procedures, 'a strict application of codes will restrain and restrict a great deal of informal, innocuous research in which students and others study groups and activities that are unproblematic' (Punch, 1998: 171). We suggest that there are four basic conditions that may justify the use of deception in a study. First, the results of the study must be of significant import. Second, participants should not be likely to suffer physical, social or psychological harm. Third, the results could not be obtained in any other way. Fourth and finally, where appropriate, debriefing should take place. If followed, these conditions should clear the way for research that might involve, *inter alia*, covert observation.

For example, a study might intend to examine the extent and antecedents of racist attitudes amongst health-care professionals[3] or football fans. The researcher would spend time gaining access to a group on a deceptive basis, perhaps even by deceptively revealing racist tendencies him/herself. In terms of contributing towards a just society, the results are clearly important. Participants would not suffer harm in the process of the research – bearing in mind issues such as the researcher not provoking behaviours, and remembering that the safety of the researcher also needs to be considered. Responses from the group in question could not be obtained in any other way, and the causes could not be inferred by simple observation, thus necessitating joining the group under false pretences. Debriefing would of course be problematic but, if handled correctly, could result in overall benefits.

This does not mean that deceptive studies should be blithely accepted by ethics committees. On the contrary, such studies need to be stringently justified according to the four conditions presented earlier. In presenting a study for approval, researchers must be aware of the all-embracing principle of respect for persons. Deception/covert research can easily violate an individual's autonomy. Nevertheless, practising deception in research does not necessarily negatively (in practical terms) affect an individual's right to self-determination. Researchers must nevertheless remain aware of the rights of potential participants, bearing in mind Zelaznik's (1993) contention that the rights of participants outweigh the rights of researchers to conduct research. By the same token, IRBs/RECs should be aware that deceptive research can be both valuable and non-maleficent.

Power and trust

Qualitative work poses potential problems for researchers, particularly when the project focuses on vulnerable groups. In such conditions, concerns regarding power, trust, confidentiality, anonymity, disclosure and so on are heightened.

Given that, in qualitative research, the researcher is the main data-collection instrument, obtaining valuable data depends on the researcher–participant relationship, as a climate of trust is a basic element for the successful data-gathering process. The ability to establish a sense of trust and maintain a fine balance between objective and empathetic involvement, and the taking of a non-judgemental stance, are key skills and abilities of qualitative researchers.

Sociological research in sport, in particular, focuses on disenfranchised and vulnerable groups. Examples of such research include Brackenridge's (2001) work on sexual abuse victims, Clarke's (1997) study of lesbian physical education teachers and Pronger's (1990) work on gay men in sport. The well-being of participants in vulnerable circumstances (e.g. children, abuse victims, gay athletes, drug-users) is of particular concern. Swain *et al.* (1998), in their work with people who have learning difficulties, note that the essentially political act of research can exploit vulnerable and powerless groups within society, further their disempowerment and contribute to their oppression. Also, when leaving the field, qualitative researchers need to reflect on the relationships that have developed, and they should consider their ethical obligations in this regard.

Researchers need to be aware of perceptions of power relationships. For example, participants may feel that, because of their particular circumstances, they cannot withdraw from a study. This may merely be because they perceive that a particular power situation exists, or because they feel coerced, or they fear some sort of sanction. Perceived sanctions may be intangible, such as a loss of 'face', embarrassment at the negative perceptions of 'drop-out' or potential loss of self-esteem. It is incumbent on researchers to provide the correct climate for participants, so that they feel empowered.

One of the key ethical issues in ethnographic research is how participants are represented and what their rights are in the research process. Even such an apparently straightforward convention using pseudonyms to name informants in ethnographic research raises further ethical dilemmas. Do the participants prefer such names? How much say do interviewees have in the overall research process? Should interviewees view final interview transcripts and quotes? If participants disagree with a researcher's interpretation of events, who has the final say? These issues point to a broader concern in terms of the relationships formed within research.

Confidentiality, anonymity and identifiers

Assurances of confidentiality are commonplace in research proposals and in information sheets given to potential research participants. We noted in Chapter 5, however, that such assurances are often (unintentionally) misleading. Without playing semantic games, researchers must recognise that the insistence on a confidentiality clause is not an offer of unassailable privacy when applied to research contexts, and simply say what we mean, that anonymity will be assured.

It is our contention that researchers often conflate and confuse the terms anonymity and confidentiality. As we saw in Chapter 5, strictly speaking, confidentiality means that the researcher will not share the elicited information with anyone, in any way. This is of course nonsense in research contexts, where dissemination is central to the process. If researchers ensure confidentiality, they cannot publish or present the data at all. Rather, what is meant of course is that anonymity should be assured, not confidentiality *per se*. Confidentiality does of course apply in other contexts, such as sports psychology support and consultancy, or coaching situations, or when obtaining psychometric test scores. Whatever pressures are applied by coaches and others for such information to be revealed, these must be resisted unless written authorisation from the client is received (Biddle *et al.*, 1992; Sachs, 1993), and it should be noted that:

> Conventionally in qualitative research the conditions under which consent is negotiated for access to and the use of data are those of openness, anonymity, or confidentiality. These are usually recommended to enable researchers to achieve certain purposes.
>
> (Tickle, 2002: 44)

Brackenridge (2001) defends a decision to 'never tell', explicitly stating that she would rather face contempt of court charges than reveal her sources. Sugden (1995) takes a similar line in his discussion of three fieldwork cases of moral conflict and personal hazard. When investigating boxing subcultures in Northern Ireland, Sugden came face to face with an IRA gunman whom they had caught inadvertently on videotape. The IRA operative demanded the tape and, when this was at first refused, put a revolver to the researcher's head. Of course this potentially enabled the researcher to identify the terrorist to the police. That he did not so do, Sugden notes, still troubles him. His justification of this inaction (independent of it rendering the research impossible to complete) was that in Northern Ireland there was an unwritten code that politics and boxing were not to be mixed: politics was to be left *outside* the gym. It is not clear that his identification would have stood up in a court of law. Nevertheless, he asserts that 'never tell' is the hardest rule for ethnographers to keep. Ultimately, his position embodies a utilitarian justification (though he does not make this explicit): telling may endanger all ethnographers, which would in turn have greater social dis-benefits. The calculation would be a difficult one to undertake but would prove an interesting case study in research ethics courses.

A fictitious example may illustrate this. A researcher is attempting to investigate reasons for teenage drop-out in gymnastics. S/he agrees with all participants that their anonymity will be respected, and that any unwanted and personal disclosures to her/him by participants will be treated as strictly confidential. So, what does s/he do if a participant reveals that her/his reason for thinking about leaving the sport was persistent, ongoing and serious sexual abuse by her/his coach? What is the researcher, who is not a trained counsellor, to do? Without going into the specific courses of action open to the researcher (which are not relevant here), it is clear that the researcher must do something. That is, s/he is morally obliged to act. In this case, there is a justification for overriding confidentiality in the interest of the athlete concerned, and indeed other athletes. While the example is a difficult one, or where a variety of arguments have weight, it serves to illustrate that confidentiality should not be considered absolute in principle.

Generally speaking, however, anonymity, confidentiality and privacy are cornerstones in solidifying the relationship between researcher and partici-pant in the qualitative research process. Trust is implicit in the relationship, and must be maintained unless there are exceptional circumstances as described above. Where possible, the emergence of instances such as those which arose in the gymnastics example should be identified in advance and appropriate measures put in place. Ethics committees are more likely to approve projects that provide evidence of such planning than if a response to situations is perceived as *ad hoc*.

An assurance of anonymity has an inverse relationship with requests for openness, in that the more forthcoming the researcher wants the participant to be, the more stringent assurances of anonymity need to be. Put differently, if you want a participant to speak openly and honestly, s/he needs to trust you. Trust is central to Tickle's conditions and qualitative researchers need to ensure that trust is present and maintained.

The crux of the anonymity and confidentiality issue is to safeguard against the invasion of privacy by assurance of anonymity. What we actually mean, of course, is that we will only disclose results in a manner in which partici-pants cannot be identified. Safeguarding the identity of participants is often more difficult than it seems at first. Some attempts at anonymity in pub-lished research are superficial and inadequate. For example, an article might state that, in a psychological intervention programme, the batsman with the highest average on the Australian cricket tour to India was prone to crises of confidence. Leaving aside professional obligations between the psychologist and the client and focusing purely on the publication/dissemination issue, it would clearly not need a particularly good detective to find out who the batsman concerned was. This topic has been the focus for recent discussion about the boundaries of professionalism in sports psychology (Andersen, 2005; Jones, 2005). Clearly the role boundaries are unclear for the psychologist, who is at one and the same time researcher, consultant, confidant and at the same time facing a double bind of commitment to client A (individual athlete) or B (coach/team). Heyman and Andersen (1998) report the field story of a psychologist who, on being informed that Client A (athlete) was gay, leaked the information to Client B (coach), who excluded the athlete from the team. There cannot be much clearer examples of the culpable overriding of confidentiality than this. Other failings are often far less clear.

In research writing, richness of description (and subsequent analysis) depends on providing sufficient detail and context to the reader. Identifiers and characteristics (the detail referred to earlier) make anonymity difficult, so the temptation is to delete them from the reports. On the other hand, they provide context to the findings and the discussion, so to leave them out renders the work sterile and perhaps lacking relevance. As Sparkes (1998) has pointed out, first, it is difficult to disguise somebody when they have had a high profile in a specific sport. Second, there is the tension between the need for thick description to provide a holistic portrayal and context on the one hand, and preserving anonymity on the other. So the dilemma is that good qualitative case studies require 'thick description', and the better this is, the more identifiable the participant becomes. It is a fine line to tread and perhaps we need to again return to Zelaznik's (1993) injunction to give precedence to the rights of the participant. For example, in a case study approach, Fishwick (1990) had to select very broad categories for the origin of quotes (such as female, upper management) rather than specific job titles to protect the identity of the respondents in the specific organisations.

Consider a further example, from a recent research project. In a study on motivation for participation in dangerous sports, one of the authors was faced with a situation where he could not use a particular quote from a participant without revealing their identity. At least, it could have been nominally withheld, but the description is of such a nature that anyone who had the inclination could simply type in a few key words in an internet search engine to reveal the participant's identity.[4]

We produce the particular scenario here, with explicit, active consent from the research participant, Clyde Aikau. In response to a question about any personal spiritual element involved in big wave surfing, he told the following story:

> You know, the Hawaiian people are very spiritual, and the creatures of the ocean are spiritually connected to my family. Like at Waimea Bay in 1986, the year that I won the Eddie.[5] I hadn't actually surfed the North Shore for three or four years. On the day of the event, I paddled out and there were these sea turtles, and something told me to follow the turtles.

I passed all the other guys and went out there. Sure enough, the biggest waves would come right to me, and it happened all day long. I looked at the turtles as being Eddie, my brother Eddie. It was real spiritual for us.

The aim of reproducing his quote here is that it is unique to him, but the issue goes further than that in its implications regarding anonymity. For not only is the story unique in that it only applies to Clyde Aikau, but it is ubiquitous in the lore of big wave surfing, and has been published in several forms, including the current contest promotional literature. To depersonalise this particular story would be to rob it of its poignancy – Clyde Aikau winning the inaugural event held to commemorate the deeds of his legendary late brother, and ostensibly guided by his brother in this quest through some sort of mythical reincarnation as a sea creature.

In a situation such as the one described above, one solution to the identifier-richness dilemma would be to seek *post hoc* consent from participants. This explicitly recognises the changing, emergent nature of qualitative research. While, on the face of it, it might not be desirable to alter consent arrangements during a study, there might on the other hand be strong justifications for changes. Such changes should, of course, be cleared by the relevant ethics committees prior to negotiations with participants. It is worth mentioning that the American Psychological Association (APA), for example, recognises the potential for changes in circumstance, stating that 'Unless it is not feasible or is contraindicated, the discussion of confidentiality occurs at the outset of the relationship and thereafter as new circumstances may warrant' (APA, 2002). We concur, recognising the dynamic, emergent nature of qualitative research.

If circumstances dictate, *post hoc* permission to waive anonymity is preferable to any waiver statements on consent forms. The latter, even if passed by an ethics committee, would immediately compromise authenticity by possibly producing a different response mindset in the interviewee. Without anonymity being agreed, concern would be raised that an interviewee would perhaps calculate responses as if they were intended for public consumption. Image-building, for example, would be a temptation that may be difficult to resist.

What do researchers do if *post hoc* permission is refused? If it is just one or two interviews out of 15 to 20, then, depending on the importance of the data in question to the overall analysis, perhaps those respondents could be left out. This is to negate any possible contribution that they have made to the study by virtue of their initial acquiescence to be interviewed, however, and could be construed as insulting to the time that they put in. Essentially, this means that, effectively, the participants' time and effort have been wasted, and they might legitimately resent the inference that their contributions to the study are not deemed meaningful and valuable (Peled and Leichentritt, 2002). Moreover, it raises questions regarding design and authenticity of data, particularly if those interviews contributed to, say, the data saturation process. It is ethically and methodologically preferable to present the data in their entirety, either anonymously, or with anonymity actively waived by all participants. Again, the rights of participants, either individually or collectively, ought to outweigh the rights of the researcher.

Privacy in qualitative research

When conducting interviews, particularly those that may seek to elicit sensitive information, it is desirable to do so in a comfortable setting where privacy is assured. The reasons are obvious: participants need to feel at ease and need to be reassured that they can say whatever they wish without being overheard by third parties. Also, when considering issues of authenticity, they need to be free from any influences that might contribute to some sort of image-building or merely acquiescent (yea-saying) responses.

Participants in qualitative studies are particularly vulnerable to invasion of privacy, unwanted identification, breach of confidentiality and trust, misrepresentation and exploitation. Safeguarding privacy as well as assuring anonymity is one of the key issues within preventing harm. In using quotations, interviews in life-history research often reveal biographical details, and this makes protecting identities extremely problematic. Changing names and places is no guarantee of anonymity, and this may in any case be against the wishes of participants.

But is complete privacy always possible when rich data are being transmitted? What if an athlete (where access is notoriously difficult) wants to meet and be interviewed in a semi-private place (for example, a stadium locker room)? Or what if a child's parents insist on being present during the interview process? In both cases, the researcher needs to make a judgement about authenticity of data. Will the presence of others (athletes passing through the locker room; or the parents potentially acting coercively) affect the veracity of responses? Privacy should be striven for, but it cannot always be guaranteed. Authenticity of data is however critically important, and a *post hoc* judgement might have to be made about whether or not the data ought to be used. So, if a participant demands that an interview take place in a non-private setting, the researcher can go ahead, but judgement should be carefully exercised as to whether outside influences have affected the process and the participant's responses. In a slightly different context, Sparkes (1998: 80) has said 'Stories, then, can provide powerful insights into the lived experiences of others in ways that can inform, awaken and disturb readers . . .'. As qualitative researchers, it is our business to hear, analyse and synthesise these stories. To not hear them because of an uncritical acceptance of privacy requirements would be counterproductive. Likewise, to distort them by disregarding authenticity would be irresponsible.

Beneficence

Peled and Leichentritt (2002) contend that providing participants with some research-related benefits is a minimal requirement. In much feminist work and action research, a basic premise is that participants should emerge from research with greater benefits than which they entered the project. Such 'values direct us to go beyond fairness in those with our relationship with research participants, and to use the research to contribute to personal and social empowerment of vulnerable and disenfranchised groups' (Peled and Leichentritt, 2002: 148). For example, Clarke's (1997) research on lesbian physical education teachers provides an opportunity for the participants to tell their story, and reveals something of their lived experience, which serves to challenge the oppressive structures that 'force' them to conceal their lesbian identities. By making the women the subject and not the object of analysis, she does much to make these encounters more accessible, helpful, empowering and respectful for lesbians.

Payments to research participants are not as common in qualitative work as they are in quantitative work, such as clinical trials. However, remunerating participants is becoming increasingly common and might be welcomed by participants in qualitative studies, particularly if they are financially disadvantaged. Without repeating the general norms set out in Chapter 4, we shall make some cursory remarks in relation to this in qualitative work in particular. Remunerating participants is, as we have seen, not without ethical import. Generally speaking, payments should not be such that they constitute a temptation to disregard any risks associated with participation, or that they affect a person's ability to make a rational judgement about participation where they will form an undue inducement (Jago and Bailey, 2001). Another perspective is that payment is deemed excessive if it exceeds the equivalent of a minimum wage for the time spent by a participant on a project (Shephard, 2002). Either way, payments should never constitute coercion.

At present, beneficence is an issue on which researchers will need to make individual value judgements. Ethics committees dominated by the biomedical tradition are unlikely to insist on benefits for participants, as they will probably view increased knowledge as a sufficient good in itself. What they might question, however, is the notion of external validity (generalisability) or the lack thereof (see Sparkes, 1992, for a discussion of this issue). This is a debate too specific for the purposes of this chapter. The reason for raising the issue here, though, is that ethics committees nowadays concern themselves with more than ethical matters, and both the design and 'value' of projects may be debated. In the context of committees influenced by the positivist tradition, qualitative researchers would be well advised to prepare reasons that advance the claims of the authenticity, credibility, trustworthiness and value of their work. This will assist in accelerating the education process, whereby ethics committees need to be more cognisant of issues faced by qualitative researchers.

Diverse and emergent issues

Given the diverse approaches to qualitative work in exercise, health and sports sciences it would be neither feasible nor desirable to provide set ethical guidelines to cover all eventualities. Qualitative studies in these spheres range from structured interviews, content analysis and pre-determined sample sizes at one extreme, to unstructured sports ethnographies. Access to research populations is sometimes through institutional gatekeepers, sometimes through informal contacts or snowballing. Given this range, it would be unlikely that any code of ethics could address key dilemmas in a meaningful way. If a code could address all the issues, it would probably be too general to be of any practical use. If it were specific, it would not cover the diverse range of issues confronting qualitative researchers. The same applies to research ethics for qualitative researchers. It is not always possible to identify and quantify risks in qualitative work. Unsolicited self-reflection is one such issue. To ensure that ethical problems that emerge during the conduct of research are dealt with, researchers need to establish a mechanism of referral at the outset. This will not necessarily be the same as the 'oversight' system demanded by some biomedical ethics dominated committees. The oversight model might in fact be inappropriate for some types of qualitative research, particularly those that require privacy, anonymity and the establishment of trust. Nevertheless, researchers and committees should identify the means to report ethical issues, and the means to solve them or receive guidance about them.

In support of the concept of qualitative research ethics as an ongoing process, Swain *et al.* (1998) hold that qualitative studies are inherently fraught with ethical dilemmas that cannot be predicted at the outset. They argue that there is a need for ethical guidelines that focus on the research process and which complement codes concerned with the planning stage. This frames ethics as a continuous process of decision-making.

Playing the game

Despite problems with setting concrete guidelines for ethics in research, investigators still need to get approval from IRBs/RECs before they can collect data. At present, the highly structured, strongly regulated, bureaucratic and ubiquitous IRB/REC system is the only game in town. This places qualitative researchers at a disadvantage relative to quantitative investigators when it comes to ethics review and approval of projects. It is likely that, as qualitative research gains credence in the research community, IRBs/RECs will become more sensitised to the design, methods of data collection and analysis of qualitative work. Qualitative researchers can assist this educative process by understanding how IRBs/RECs make their decisions and then structure their research proposals to facilitate approval. Qualitative researchers are thus advised to, *inter alia*: anticipate problems and think imaginatively and prospectively about solving them; seek qualified advice before submitting potentially problematic proposals to IRBs/RECs; incorporate a monitoring, review and referral process into their proposals; make sure that they have a strong, defensible research design, with a cogent argument and a clear decision trail; be able to give a simple, clear account of the problem and why it is worth investigating; be able to give a reasoned account of the methods of data collection and analysis, including emergent issues and how they might be dealt with; have some equivalent to generalisability, for example that a thick, rich account of a particular setting will produce an understanding that will have value in other settings; and demonstrate an appreciation of the rights of individuals and groups that may participate in the study.

Conclusion

Research in exercise, health and sports sciences has historically been dominated by quantitative methods and traditions, and the positivistic predilections that typically support them. This is changing, but it is not clear that the mechanisms for evaluating the ethical merits of studies are keeping pace. The methods employed in qualitative work mean that researchers face different ethical problems compared to their quantitative colleagues. Researchers and ethics committees need to be aware of the differences, and projects must be planned and presented to committees accordingly. The wide range of methods in inductive approaches makes it difficult to formulate specific guidelines for ethical conduct. Nevertheless, qualitative researchers should attempt to foresee both obvious and emerging ethical problems when they plan their research. Having done so, they should set support, monitoring and reporting mechanisms in place. While we have argued that some ethical principles are not carved in stone, researchers ought to follow the overarching principle of respect for persons. When confronted with ethical dilemmas, the rights of the participants should be seen as outweighing the rights of the researcher to conduct research.

8   Research ethics and vulnerable populations

Children and other 'vulnerable populations'[1]

While there has not been widespread discussion of ethical aspects of research on children in exercise and sports settings[2] the topic is not a new one in health care and medical ethics (Nicholson, 1986; Brazier and Lobjoit, 1991; Alderson, 1992; Kopelman, 2000; Spriggs, 2004). The omission is instructive in itself. Yet there is an increasing literature in the fields of the natural sciences of exercise and sports regarding children's anatomy and physiology, developmental studies and kinanthropometry. It should be clear that children form the largest category of what is typically referred to as a 'vulnerable population' in research design and research ethics. In this chapter we will focus on them for this reason, though it should be clear that many of the considerations will apply – *mutatis mutandis* – to other vulnerable populations as well. Nevertheless, we amplify our remarks where appropriate to other vulnerable populations. One main aim of the chapter is to make the reader (further) aware of the various professional guidelines that exist to govern research in this area: the World Medical Association (WMA) Declaration of Helsinki, on the one hand, and the guidance offered by the British Medical Association (BMA), the Royal College of Paediatric and Child Health (RCPCH; formerly the British Paediatric Association [BPA]), and the Council for International Organizations of Medical Sciences (CIOMS).[3] We go on to highlight some theoretical difficulties in their application and, at the end of the chapter, conceptually challenge the labelling 'vulnerable populations' itself.

Vulnerability and trust

Why ought we to take a given population and treat them in a special way? Thus far we have illustrated a variety of contexts and issues in order to elaborate various duties and virtues of researchers bearing in mind the rights of participants across the research spectrum. For what reasons might we appear to go against a general ethical norm of treating all persons equally? One very clear reason can be taken from Aristotle's writings on equality. For

Aristotle makes the key point that to treat persons with equality does not entail that we treat them all in the same manner. On first sight this appears contradictory. Closer inspection reveals that it is not, for his formal principle of equality of treatment reads: 'treat equals equally, treat unequals unequally' (Aristotle, 1998). Is there something about a particular group or population that makes them unequal, so that they thereby merit different treatment? It is widely thought that there are groups of our societies who, by their very nature, are more easily exploited or harmed than are others. For this reason, it is thought, they deserve special consideration. Such people are deemed in the literature to belong to a 'vulnerable population'. Their unequal vulnerability places an obligation on researchers to treat them differently and this obligation or duty is widely evidenced in formal codes of conduct for research, in Institutional Research Board (IRB) or Research Ethics Committee (REC) procedures and checklists, and in the practices of researchers from across the research spectrum in exercise, health and sports sciences research.

Writing almost two decades ago Mitford (1988) noted a troubling equivocation by the WMA who, in 1961, had argued that prisoners 'being captive groups, should not be used as the subject of experiments'. She notes that the recommendation was never formally adopted by the WMA because of the opposition of American doctors. She then goes on to note:

> 'Pertinax' writing in the *British Medical Journal* for January 1963, says 'I am disturbed that the World Medical Association is now hedging on its clause about using criminals as experimental behaviour. The American influence has been at work on its suspension.' He adds wistfully, 'One of the nicest American scientists I know was heard to say, "Criminals in our penitentiaries are fine experimental material – and much cheaper than chimpanzees."' I hope [Mitford adds] the chimpanzees don't come to hear of this.
>
> (Mitford, 1988: 189)

Clearly, Mitford's writing represents a picture that is more than three decades old. Research governance procedures, as we saw in Chapter 3, have moved on very considerably since then and not least in relation to vulnerable populations, whether captive (as in the case of prisoners) or others. Notwithstanding this, our understanding of why researchers are not merely justified but rather obliged to give them special consideration requires a further exemplification of the notions of autonomy and paternalism. We saw in Chapter 4 how the issue of informed consent hinged on a proper appreciation of these significant moral concepts. They play a key role in our understanding of how to treat vulnerable populations too, and also how we understand that vulnerability. The perception that those belonging to vulnerable populations cannot meet the complex conditions of informed consent drives the paternalism present in the duty to give them special attention. It is not dissimilar from a general legal principle of a duty of care.

It is important to note how this paternalistic stance in respect of vulnerable populations connects with what is often considered to be the first principle of medical ethics. It is famously captured in the Latin phrase: *primum non nocere*. This is traditionally translated as 'first, do no harm'. It is often formulated as a moral principle: non-maleficence discussed in Chapter 2.

This duty is often though to be the bedrock of medical ethics, since the patient is dependent upon the medical physician in a situation that is properly characterised as one of trust (Baier, 1993; O'Neill, 2002). It is important to note that when social scientists (such as sociologists or economists) discuss the concept of trust, it is more felicitous to say that they are often talking about mere reliability or probability (McNamee, 1998). When they ask whether someone be trusted to do X, they mean no more than how likely is it that X will do Y at time T. If, however, we understand trust as an *ethical* and not merely a social concept, we must recognise that one of its preconditions is the notion of vulnerability (Baier, 1993). To trust someone, in this sense, is to be *entrusted* with a certain power. Those who enjoy our trust in this sense are those who, in some way, can be harmed by us. This is how Baier highlights the relations between the vulnerability of the truster and the power of the trusted:

> . . . look at the variety of sorts of goods or things one values or cares about, which can be left or put within the striking powers of others, and the variety of ways we can let or leave others 'close' enough to what we value to be able to harm it. Then we can look at various reasons we might have for wanting or accepting such closeness of those with power to harm us, and for confidence that they will not use this power.
>
> (Baier, 1993: 100)

What Baier does not explore, but may have been close to the surface, is the very idea of trust's relation to 'confidence' in the older sense of that word whereby one might say 'I'll bring you into my confidence'; what may be said or done, for example, may be privileged or secret, and one places one's trust in another to retain that status.

This is apposite for our understanding of the mechanisms of research in exercise, health and sports, which must be carried out for, on and with other human beings. Across society, generally speaking, many of our achievements require the coordination of effort by many persons. This is certainly true of research. In the acquisition and development of new knowledge through research – especially to gain knowledge beneficial to populations – we cannot but help to leave others in striking distance of them.

> Since the things we typically do value include such things as we cannot singlehandedly either create or sustain (our own life, health, reputation, our offspring and their well-being, as well as intrinsically shared goods such as conversation, its written equivalent, theater and other forms of

play, chamber music, market exchange, political life and so on) we must allow many other people to get into positions where they can, if they choose, injure what we care about, since those are the same positions that they must be in order to help us take care of what we care about.

(Baier, 1993: 100–1)

Two other points should be added. First, viewing trust this way helps bring up the notion of norms and expectations and their limits in a language that cannot merely be technical. Second, by so doing, Baier raises to our attention the notion of implicit trusting and the failure of contractual devices such as codes of conduct to address every eventuality. This point may be related to the notion of deontology's under-determination of the moral sphere; in avoiding harm and respecting others we are still left with a multitude of choices. We shall see that the rules regarding the ethics of research with vulnerable populations are relatively clear. Yet, in addition to these rules, the IRBs and RECs must trust that the rules will be upheld.

> We need some fairly positive and discretion-allowing term, such as 'look after' or 'show concern for' . . . We also need some specification of what good was in question to see why the intrusive, presumptuous, and pater-nalistic moves disappoint rather than meet the trust one has in such circumstances. 'Look after' and 'take care of' will have to be given a very weak sense in some cases of trust; it will be better to do this than try to construe cases where more positive care is expected of the trusted as cases of trusting them to leave alone, or merely safeguard, the entrusted valued thing.
>
> (Baier, 1993: 103)

Given that we impart to the trusted a valued thing within limits of dis-cretionary power we thereby risk abuse of such. Worse, it is open to as yet unnoticed harm of disguised ill will. This is not something to be avoided; it comes part and parcel with trust itself:

> To understand the moral risks of trust, it is important to see the special sort of vulnerability it introduces. Yet the discretionary element which introduces this special danger is essential to that which trust at its best makes possible. To elaborate Hume: 'Tis impossible to separate the chance of good from the risk of ill.'
>
> (Baier, 1993: 103, citing Hume, 1978: 497)

Given that we cannot watch over all research, the presence of efficacious rules, with powerful sanctions, acts as one institutional lever to guide right thinking in research. We shall now examine some relevant codes of conduct to see how they cater for vulnerability of research participants and subjects.

Vulnerable populations in codes of conduct

If researchers are to avoid the exploitation of the vulnerability of subjects/participants, it will be necessary to know first who might be thought of as vulnerable and what forms such exploitation might take. We will focus on the first of these issues predominantly.

One of the difficulties in generalising the nature of ethical issues with vulnerable populations is of course conceptual. We will address below some of the philosophical difficulties with the concept. But there are less deep issues too in terms of the heterogeneity of the nomenclature's reach: who is to count? There is no absolutely agreed standard. We cite here a comprehensive list of populations who fall under the title 'vulnerable'. It comes from the World Health Organization's (WHO) Research Ethics Review Committee, Checklist for Principal Investigators:

- adolescents
- children
- elderly
- pregnant women
- prisoners
- refugees
- persons with mental or behavioural disorders, and
- persons who cannot give their consent (unconscious).

There is a further category: others. Precisely who is to be defined under this category is, of course, completely unclear. This is less than helpful. But then perhaps we should observe the differential status of each of the categories that comprise the group. It is hard to imagine, in most cases, a justification for research being conducted on unconscious persons. We shall return to these problems at the end of the chapter.

The prison population is discrete and easy to identify. We might think this is the case with pregnant women too. But how do we know when we should consider an elderly patient to be vulnerable? What shall we count as a behavioural disorder? Thomas Szasz once famously argued that the category of mental illness itself was a myth – since the mind cannot be ill in the same way that the body can it is better not to refer to mental illnesses as such. And, of course, the same criticism may be applied to mental dis/order.

Perhaps another way might be to alert researchers to the considerations that might affect the appropriateness of vulnerable persons' (VP) involvement. Beyrer and Kass (2002) cite the following:

- vulnerability
- poverty
- human rights violations
- discrimination

- poor access to resources
- education
- coercion
- lack of trust.

Having set out these vulnerable populations the WHO checklist helpfully asks two key questions. What is the justification for the use of this population viz. the research questions; and what provisions have been made to avoid exploitation of these populations? This latter question goes to the heart of the matter, which we shall explore in detail in relation to the largest element of the vulnerable populations: children.

Why do research on, with and for children?

In his review article, Shephard (2002: 171) acknowledges a general norm: that care should be taken not to exploit the vulnerable in research. Recognising this norm, he expresses later a general principle: 'If the research can be conducted on a less vulnerable group, then it should be' (2002: 173). If we accept these general edicts, which are widely held, the responsibility is clearly upon researchers, therefore, to justify the inclusion of vulnerable populations as research subjects or participants.[4] Are there good reasons for conducting clinical research on children? We might consider at least three.

First, certain interesting research problems emanate from the populations themselves. So, for example, certain diseases are characteristically childhood diseases and therefore meaningful research on them needs to be conducted on children. Thus, if we want to explore the biological (and not just the cultural) reasons for the apparent obesity pandemic, we must study children.[5]

Second, there are well-known problems in extrapolating pharmacological data from adults to children due to differences between children and adults. More generally these difficulties may arise at a biological (Kopelman, 2000; Hebestreit and Bar-Or, 2005; ACSM [American College of Sports Medicine], 2006), biomechanical (Yeadon and Morlock, 1989), or psychological or socio-cultural levels. Because of such differences, for example, effects of drugs may differ (effects dangerously enhanced or paradoxically diminished – differences in pharmaco-kinetics.) Reye's Syndrome provides an instructive example. Aspirin given to children under the age of 12 can cause Reye's Syndrome, which is indicated, among other things, by severe swelling of the brain. It took some years of clinical experience before anyone realised the connection between the taking of aspirin and the occurrence of Reye's. This is a classic example of a specific age-related metabolic difference with fatal consequences, undetected because the drug had not been tested on children. Also, due to the dearth of research on children, many drugs used in treatment of children have not been tested upon them in clinical trials.

Third, research on children is necessary to determine what is normal development in order to ensure that ensuing policy, practice guidelines or treatments (RCPCH, 2000) given are appropriate (Nicholson, 1986; Kopelman, 2000). Another way of putting this justification is that conditions can only be identified as abnormal when they are seen in relation to what is normal. And this will require research on and with the relevant populations. Although these are indeed good grounds for conducting research on children, the absence of their consent, in conjunction with their vulnerability, presents important countervailing considerations.

Thus, if research is to be permitted upon non-consenting children, it is crucial that there are appropriate guidelines governing the selection of children and the conduct of the research. This is an especially important point in the current climate in which pharmaceutical companies are seeking to develop treatments for childhood diseases such as attention deficit disorder, childhood autism and more general childhood psychopathologies. Yet current guidelines, we show, generate considerable confusion.

Protecting children from being treated as 'mere' means in research

In this section we shall begin with the position enshrined in the WMA Declaration of Helsinki and show how it is at odds with guidelines offered by the BMA, the RCPCH (formerly the BPA), and CIOMS.

It is fair to observe that the WMA Declaration of Helsinki (2000) provides the backdrop against which the legitimacy of other guidelines concerning the ethical conduct of research is constrained. This is signalled in its title of course (a product of the World Medical Association). And, as would be expected, the RCPCH/BPA, for example, indicate that their guidelines are thus constrained. The WMA Helsinki Declaration prioritises the welfare of the research subject over the interests of research institutions and society more generally. Thus:

> In medical research on human subjects [sic], considerations related to the well-being of the human subject should take precedence over the interests of science and society.
> (WMA, 2000: 8; see also RCPCH, 2000: 178; CIOMS, 2002: 6)

Although not as precise, nor as strict, as might be preferred by those who wish absolutely to protect the subject, a plausible interpretation of the clause might run as follows. Within these codes, the well-being of the human subject counts for more, morally speaking, than scientific progress, for example in the form of acquisition of new knowledge. And the well-being of the subject counts for more, morally speaking, than the interests of society. This would rule out, then, utilitarian perspectives that might seek to justify researchers' duties to respect participants'/subjects' rights on the grounds of beneficent outcomes as we shall see below.

It should be stressed that, as with any code of conduct, and perhaps every piece of ethical theorising, there is scope for differences in interpretation of the clause cited above. Let us see, however, the extent to which one might find a robust ethical authority for its prescription. One obvious starting point, as noted in Chapter 2, would be the deontological writings of Kant in his 'practical imperative'. According to this, one must:

> Act in such a way that you always treat humanity, whether in your own person or in the person of any other, never simply as a means, but always at the same time as an end.
>
> (Kant, 1948 [1785]: 91)

The invocation of Kant's imperative helps to explain just what would be wrong from the moral point of view with violating the Helsinki clause. If a participant/subject is researched upon without their consent simply to promote the interests of science or society, that subject is being used as a 'mere' means, an instrument of external agency/ies (including researchers) and their ends, in violation of the imperative.

It is worth making two additional points in broad support of the Kantian imperative, for although it belongs classically to deontological theory, it has very widespread appeal in common sense. The first is that the wrongness of using other human beings as a mere means to one's own (or others') ends is a widely shared aspect of ordinary morality at a global level – note we do not say 'universally'. To be described as a person who uses others (here: research subjects) for their own ends is to be described in terms that are morally critical. A good researcher would be disturbed to learn that others viewed them in such a way. A cursory examination of the rich vocabulary that the English language supplies gives voice to moral criticism of others in the same way: for example, to describe that person as devious, disrespectful or manipulative. This is one way in which, for example, deontologists and virtue theorists, coming from radically different starting points, might easily agree on their condemnation of such conduct and character. What has been said thus far might easily apply to all research populations *ceteris paribus*. We shall now apply this thinking to vulnerable populations by way of children as research participants/subjects.

Children in health related exercise research: the case of venepuncture

It is plausibly held that all research subjects are in a position of vulnerability – they are in a condition in which they could suffer harm (Evans and Evans, 1996). This is the case even if they are capable of consenting to participate in medical research. As we have seen in Chapter 4, the relationship between researcher and participant/subject is not an 'equal' one (Alderson, 1992; Evans and Evans, 1996). The former has qualifications, high social status; the researched in these contexts are most likely to lack these or at least perceive the situation thus.

There are certain research settings, medical research notwithstanding, where issues of vulnerability may be exacerbated. Consider much of the research on exercise and obesity; may not children feel parental and other social pressures to engage in such research and at least be seen to be attempting to conform to social norms? Might it not also be the case that parents who will give proxy consent, and even the assenting child, may feel that engagement with the research will help at least lay the platform for a future slimmer self and more socially acceptable lifestyle? The exercise physiology laboratory will seem a strange and powerful location. They may easily feel obliged to conform to the researcher's wishes even before the informed consent process has been initiated. Whether this should or should not trouble researchers may not be straightforward and probably rests on the estimation of benefits and risks and the directness of these. We shall consider these aspects of risk in the research design so that they might inform (excuse the pun) informed consent processes.

The RCPCH distinguishes three categories of risk: minimal, low and high. Minimal risk includes 'using blood from a sample that has been taken as part of treatment' (2000: 177). Low risk includes 'procedures that cause brief pain or tenderness, and small bruises or scars [e.g.] . . . injections and venepuncture' (2000: 179).[6] 'High risk procedures such as lung or liver biopsy . . . are not justified for research purposes alone' (2000: 179).

As originally formulated, before an amendment which we will discuss very shortly, the RCPCH/BPA guidelines included the following clause: 'It would be unethical to submit child subjects [sic] to more than minimal risk when the procedure offers no benefit to them, or only a slight or very uncertain one' (BPA, 1992: 9). According to this original version of the guidelines, venepuncture would not be ethically defensible if the research is intended to benefit future child patients, and will not benefit the child research subject themselves. This version certainly respects the Kantian imperative discussed above, and unequivocally respects clause 5 of the WMA Helsinki Declaration discussed above. But apparently the original formulation was considered excessively restrictive and was subsequently revised as follows:

> We believe that research in which children are submitted to more than minimal risk with only slight, uncertain or no benefit to themselves deserves serious ethical consideration.
>
> (RCPCH, 2000: 179)

Thus research involving venepuncture, for example, is now thought permissible having previously been deemed unethical. The revised version is surely vulnerable to the charge of being excessively permissive. It now omits to forbid research in which child subjects are used merely as means for the benefit of future children. Much health-related research, such as physiological studies on exercise and obesity, or asthma, or even on high-intensity exercise, would seem to fall into this category. Not only does this transgress the Kantian imperative sketched above, but it also seems to violate clause 5 of the WMA Helsinki Declaration, which forbids research that places the interests of other parties over the well-being of the researched.

For the assessment of physical activity, blood lactate is normally taken in children and adults via a capillary sample from the ear lobe or finger. Sometimes taking serial samples of blood from the same site can prove painful but this may not trouble researchers even where an alternative can-nula approach could be taken. A review of some recent exercise physiology research, however, throws up examples where venepuncture has been used in non-therapeutic research (Martinez and Haymes, 1992; Tolfrey *et al.*, 1999; Alten and Mariscalco, 2003; Tsalis *et al.*, 2004).[7] It is questionable whether this research – which doubtless will have moved through IRBs/RECs as was relevant – is ethically justifiable, even where it has been legitimated by research governance procedures. It is hard to see how it can be in a child's best interests to be a research subject in these circumstances, undergoing venepuncture for the benefit of future children. And in fact it seems plaus-ible to regard it to be contrary to a child's best interests to undergo such non-therapeutic procedures.

In defence of the RCPCH/BPA guidelines, one aspect is particularly note-worthy. The guidelines permit children themselves to determine whether an intervention presents a low or a minimal risk (RCPCH, 2000: 178–9). However, this can only apply when children are capable of making such a determination. Moreover, it seems reasonable to point out that even older children may not be capable of making such an assessment until after the intervention has been carried out (e.g. if they have not previously experi-enced the intervention). So the concerns raised here against the RCPCH guidelines seem to stand. We turn now to the CIOMS guidelines.

CIOMS guideline 9 focuses on risk to subjects unable to consent – includ-ing children. Guideline 9: 'Special limitations on risk when research involves individuals who are not capable of giving informed consent' states:

> When there is ethical and scientific justification to conduct research with individuals incapable of giving informed consent, the risk from research interventions that do not hold out the prospect of direct benefit for the individual subject should be no more likely and not greater than the risk attached to routine medical or psychological examination of such per-sons. Slight or minor increases above such risk may be permitted when there is an overriding scientific or medical rationale for such increases and when an ethical review committee has approved them.
>
> (CIOMS, 2002)

Guideline 9 holds explicitly that research on subjects, with a certain level of risk, is justified even when the subject won't directly benefit from the research. Two levels of risk are specified: (a) a low-risk standard and (b) a standard slightly above this.

The 'low-risk' standard says the research on non-competent children can be justified provided the risk of harm to the subject is not greater than risk of harm incurred during routine medical procedures. Hence this guideline seems to endorse research on incompetent children which: (a) does not directly benefit the child; (b) may include risk of harm ('low risk'). This guideline may lead to a violation of clause 5 of the WMA Declaration of Helsinki. Unless the child has an untreatable condition, it is not clear how it can be in the child's interests to permit them to be used merely as a means for the benefit of future patients. Note too that the CIOMS clause permits such research even if the risks of harm to the non-consenting subject are in fact greater than a low risk, e.g. if they involve 'slight or minor increases above [low] risk' (2002: 30).

The distinction between non-therapeutic and therapeutic research with respect to children

With the exception of the most recent WMA Declaration of Helsinki, the guidelines discussed above each seems to presuppose the possibility of drawing a robust distinction between therapeutic and non-therapeutic research. Thus, for example, recall the RCPCH statement quoted above: 'We therefore support the premise that research that is of no intended benefit to the child subject is not necessarily unethical or illegal' (RCPCH, 2000: 178). The clear implication here is that some research can be of direct benefit to the child participant/subject. But such a distinction has been subject to criticism (Alderson, 1992; Evans and Evans, 1996; Edwards, 2000; Spriggs, 2004). Critics point out that the research context is one in which the primary aim is extension of knowledge, not the well-being of the research subject (though of course this should not be neglected). So, contrary to the guidelines discussed above, it is far from clear that a robust distinction between therapeutic and non-therapeutic research can be articulated.

The implications of this for our discussion are as follows. Suppose it is allowed that there is a distinction between therapeutic and non-therapeutic research. Two positions concerning the ethics of research on non-consenting children are coherent ones. A first permits such research providing it is therapeutic in nature (providing the subject directly benefits). A second forbids such research on grounds that there is no direct benefit to the subject. But if it is accepted that the distinction between therapeutic and non-therapeutic research is spurious, then the two positions are no longer available. If one shows non-therapeutic research on children incapable of giving consent to be morally objectionable, one thereby shows all such research on non-consenting children to be morally objectionable. Our discussion has refrained from advancing this radical claim. Instead we have queried the defensibility of research on non-consenting children, which is of no benefit to them (is non-therapeutic), and which involves the experience of some discomfort or pain on their part. As shown, current guidelines seem to permit the possibility of such research. We have argued that such a permissive stance is not consistent with clause 5 of the WMA Declaration of Helsinki.

From paternalism to empowerment?

Some commentators observe a shift in emphasis away from the exclusion of vulnerable populations from the research sample where there is no direct benefit to be gained to a position where equity considerations might require that researchers consider the inclusion of such populations in their research. The shift in the salience of moral terrain is one from paternalism to justice. One might reasonably ask how the ethical stance of exclusion of such populations for reasons of their protection can be justified. It appears that this may be considered a new norm whereby the inclusion of vulnerable populations was desirable or perhaps even obligatory.

We began the chapter with a discussion of how it is that research with/on these populations might be desirable. We noted how, in certain circumstances, it was epistemically necessary to research that population given its uniqueness in terms of the research problem. Moreover, it can be argued that if the benefits of researching that population are considered properly, the burdens of that research ought also to fall – proportionately – to that population. This is a clear justice-driven consideration. A widely shared intuition about justice in the Western world may be expressed in the following norm: benefits and burdens ought to be distributed fairly among members of a community or society. Irrespective, therefore, of their status as 'vulnerable', pregnant women, or intellectually disabled populations, or minority ethnic groups might be expected to participate in research. Thus guideline 12 of the CIOMS policy reads:

> Groups or communities to be invited to be subjects of research should be selected in such a way that the burdens and benefits of the research will be equitably distributed. The exclusion of groups or communities that might benefit from study participation must be justified.
>
> (CIOMS, 2002)

Before leaping, however, to the radical conclusion that the pendulum of power had swung entirely from paternalistic protectionism to empowerment, they offer in guideline 13 the following strong caution:

> Special justification is required for inviting vulnerable individuals to serve as research subjects [sic] and, if they are selected, the means of protecting their rights and welfare must be strictly applied.
>
> (CIOMS, 2002)

This is one aspect then where extrapolation from child-considerations to other vulnerable populations is not straightforward. Perhaps none are as plausible as we have assumed. This guideline stands in the starkest contrast to the politicisation of the Disability Rights Movement (DRM). This movement has argued that allowing others to be their voice has reinforced a culture of dependency and has exposed them to misrepresentation. The goals of authentic representation and empowerment are captured in the memorable phrase, which is the title of a leading book in the field of disability studies, 'nothing about us without us' (Charlton, 1998). Charlton writes, with a large measure of rhetorical flourish, of the implications of this research tradition:

> The DRM's demand for control is the essential theme that runs through all its work, regardless of political-economic or cultural differences. Control has universal appeal for DRM activists because their needs are everywhere conditioned by a dependency born of powerlessness, poverty, degradation, and institutionalisation. This dependency saturated with paternalism, begins with the onset of disability and continues until death.
>
> (Charlton, 1998: 3)

One can find precisely the same kind of empowerment vocabulary in other areas of research related to minority or excluded populations who do not strictly fall into the category of vulnerable populations set out by the WHO. See, for example, the issue of whether white researchers ought to investigate issues of racism generally (Cashmore and Troyna, 1981; Lawrence, 1981; Rex 1981; Cashmore, 1982) and Asians being studied by white middle-class men in particular (Carrington *et al.*, 1987; Raval, 1989). Precisely who, then, ought to count as vulnerable if taking the WHO list as authoratative is not without problems? Beyrer and Kass's (2002) list set out above might look to some to be to open to be operational. More specifically, Stone (2003) notes that the economically and the educationally disadvantaged ought also be given special consideration. Given that IRBs/RECs cannot (nor would they wish to) police every piece of research, it is clear that the erection of the category 'vulnerable' itself may be thought to be problematic.

The ambiguity of 'vulnerable' as a concept

Having set out in some detail important considerations regarding the category 'vulnerable populations' we shall, somewhat paradoxically, observe the fact that in the literature there seems to be a challenge about the efficacy of the concept itself. Noting that the history of the concept can be traced back to the Belmont Report (see Chapter 3), Levine *et al.* (2004) offer three worthy arguments that may undermine the importance of considering vulnerable populations.

First they argue that, as conventionally understood, the category includes 'virtually all potential human subjects [sic]' (2004: 46). They may overstate their case here – and we have seen how the WHO categories are helpful if not exhaustive. As an alternative they cite the 2002 WMA guidelines to the effect that the economically and medically disadvantaged are to be recognised as requiring special attention. Likewise, more specific are the CIOMS guidelines, which include subordinate members of hierarchical groups. One point to be drawn from these inconsistencies has already been sketched in Chapter 3: who are the proper sources of ethical authority when jurisdiction is unclear? And they argue, moreover, that a focus on vulnerable populations may draw us away from a more significant concern over other ethically problematic aspects of research. This objection may be dealt with fairly swiftly by the reminder that addressing demographic data that enable us to identify vulnerable populations is only one of a number of important ethical considerations we should undertake. Their third point is both philosophically and sociologically acute. We must be wary as researchers, teachers of research ethics or research ethics reviewers to avoid the stereotyping of research participants based on one characteristic, or a limited set of characteristics. What follows from this is that we should be wary of simply assuming that membership of a certain group or category necessarily renders all from that category or group vulnerable or indeed a legitimate voice for that population.

A further and deeper consideration surfaces from ontological quarters: is not vulnerability the name for the human condition? Are we not vulnerable by nature? Philosophers from Descartes onwards have made observations about morbidity and the human estate, and Hobbes's recognition that even the most powerful are vulnerable to deadly assault in their sleep, most famously canonised this point.

Must we throw the baby out with the bath water? Having got this far should we reject the very idea that vulnerable populations require special consideration in research? We think not. But we must observe one further critical distinction: that between closely related concepts of vulnerability and susceptibility. Kottow puts it particularly well:

> Vulnerability is an essential attribute of mankind to be acknowledged, whereas susceptibility is a specific and accidental condition to be diagnosed and treated. Susceptible individuals have already suffered harm, they are no longer intact and are vulnerable to potential injury, they have fallen from the state of integrity to that of damaged individuality – as a chipped Sèvres vase is no longer vulnerable but damaged –. The main importance of this distinction is that vulnerability must resort to additional ethical support to gain respect and protection, whereas damaged beings are in need of repair, restoration, remedial treatment.
>
> (Kottow, 2004: 284)

The claims vulnerability makes upon us as researchers are therefore not to be cast aside because we are worried about conceptual inflation, nor because we cannot distinguish among the different levels of vulnerability, but because of a point, made most clearly by Macklin (2003). She argues quite simply that what concerns us about vulnerability is the possibility for exploitation. In itself exploitation is repugnant and to exploit those who are for a host of reasons lacking the powers properly to defend themselves against it is particularly culpable. This is what fuels the outrage that ensued after the Tuskegee experiments, as we saw in Chapter 1, where human subjects were impregnated with syphilis for the development of research in medical science.

A point sometimes made in relation to the too-casual usage of examples from Nazi Germany pertains, too, to the Tuskegee case. We endorse and hope to have avoided indulgence in our exemplification of research wrongs in this chapter and in others. Fairchild and Bayer write:

> The past decade has demonstrated that the charge of 'Tuskegee' is extremely effective in riveting public attention, but just as research demands of its practitioners that they adhere to standards of moral responsibility, challenges to research carry with them certain moral obligations. Those who would use Tuskegee to indict research efforts bear responsibility for how they deploy the legacy of that awful historical episode.
>
> While Tuskegee can stimulate productive reflection on questions of social justice, its reckless invocation risks derailing serious and sustained discussion of the dilemmas posed by research with vulnerable populations. Ironically, it can also make current research abuses pale in comparison to the historical syphilis study, thus minimizing their gravity. The abuse of Tuskegee has consequences not only for present discussion, but also for the past. It threatens to rob Tuskegee of its unique value and meaning. It misuses the memory of the 399 African American men whose most basic rights were violated for 40 years. In so doing, it diminishes the significance of their suffering.
>
> (Fairchild and Bayer, 1999: 919)

We hope that their reminder serves as an eloquent warning as much to research mentors and teachers of research ethics as it does to researchers themselves in exercise, health and sports sciences.

Conclusion

There will always be developments in the regulatory mechanisms of research ethics with regard to vulnerable populations. Whether we can expect harmonisation is quite another matter. Given the conflict between the BMA, RCPCH/BPA and CIOMS guidelines on the one hand, and the Helsinki Declaration on the other, some statement from these organisations on this conflict is urgently needed. For, as mentioned above, it is commonly assumed that the WMA Declaration provides a background that all ethically defensible guidelines concerning research on human subjects must not transgress. Yet, as we have shown, at least three current sets of guidelines seem to permit transgressions of a key clause of it.

We have briefly charted some movements between paternalistic exclusion from research to aspects of inclusion and empowerment. A further comment, however, is required with respect to the moral vocabulary of the ethical response. While the benefits and burdens of research with, for and on these populations will be variously interpreted by IRBs/RECs, and by the communities themselves, one feature of virtue ethics requires highlighting here. It is unlikely that any IRB/REC could be sensitive to every vulnerable participant/subject in its ethical deliberations. Since this is the case, it is incumbent on teachers of research ethics and, more significantly, research mentors, to be role-models and to develop research cultures that respect fully the potential for exploitation that arises in relation to research with, on or for those who are particularly vulnerable to it.

9 Does one size fit all?

Ethics in transcultural research

The commonly applied concept of informed consent, as discussed in Chapter 4, is essentially a Western notion, rooted as it is in the foundation of individual autonomy. Yet is this conception of autonomy universally accepted? If it is not, ought our applications of research ethics to be subtly revised in order to be more context sensitive, while still retaining such widespread and important elements as beneficence, justice and respect for persons? We will argue that while we do not want to slide down the slippery slope towards ethical relativism, researchers, ethics committees and regulatory bodies should think carefully about whether or not currently accepted models of ethics are universally applicable. Indeed, we will argue that they are not and, further, that considerations such as 'community involvement' in decision-making are not necessarily incompatible with individualised respect for persons. Moreover, we will argue that respect for persons is not confined to acknowledging autonomy and may require an understanding and appreciation of the values of societies to which individuals belong. We contend that the uncritical application of 'ready-made' models of research ethics in all situations is flawed, not only ethically, but methodologically as well.

The globalisation of research ethics

The Western notion of research ethics and the attendant regulatory systems can be characterised as a growth industry. Increasing regulation, publication of abuses in research, fear of litigation, global interdependence in research funding and, not least, globalisation of multiple aspects of society, have resulted in research ethics processes being applied to situations where such considerations were previously absent or ignored.

The globalisation of research ethics is not surprising, as it mirrors internationalisation in communications, travel, knowledge exchange and trade. Indeed, it could be said that the development model that is spreading is the dominant Western industrialisation one, and this Western dominance is also reflected in the prevailing research ethics model. Putting a negative slant on this dominance, Kuczeweski and McCruden (2001) have contended that 'much of medical ethics suffers from the individualistic bias of the dominant culture and political tradition of the United States'. More worryingly, French (1987: 18) asserts the view that 'The models of social science are justifications for the world capitalist system and the hegemony of the United States.'

Unfortunately, globalisation in many areas has not been accompanied by a democratisation of response in the distribution of wealth. In 1900, the richest 20 per cent of the world's population were nine times richer than the poorest 20 per cent. By 1997 this ratio had increased to over 70 times. Absolute poverty has also increased and, of 52 million people who die each year, 18 million die of infectious and parasitic diseases, many of these in the developing world. Life expectancy is much lower in developing countries and health spending is correspondingly poorer. There are thus widening disparities between the rich and the poor, between and within countries (Benatar, 2002).

Recent decades, though, have witnessed the emergence of ideologies of public social conscience, and this has resulted in a growth of research to address issues of inequality of, for example, health provision. The emergent model of research ethics in these situations has been the application of the Western biomedical ethics model. In some cases this has been the voluntary application of the Council for International Organizations of Medical Sciences (CIOMS) guidelines. In other cases, researchers are bound by regulations and must adhere to certain predetermined procedures regarding informed consent and ethical review of the project, regardless of the location of the project (Dawson and Kass, 2005). It is this inflexibility that we believe is potentially damaging, both in terms of disrespect for prevailing cultural values and in terms of potentially negatively affecting the validity of studies.

Literacy, language and comprehension

Perhaps the most obvious place to start to evaluate the negative aspects of the naïve application of Western research ethics is to consider the use of language, specifically as used in the informed consent process. As mentioned in Chapter 4, there is sometimes a presumption that achieving written consent is a necessary and sufficient condition for ethical research to be conducted. This is, of course, prejudicial as much valuable research takes place in illiterate societies. Some of the most urgently needed health and medical research, must, of necessity, be sited in impoverished communities, where literacy levels may be low or non-existent. For example, the prevalence of certain medical conditions (such as HIV), or the absence of certain health-care provisions (such as inoculations) may predispose research to be undertaken in certain communities. Similarly, in exercise and sports sciences, valuable research on either physical activity or health may take place with an illiterate marathon runner from an impoverished rural area, or in rural communities where a certain type of diet is worthy of study.

Clearly, in conditions such as those sketched above, where participants are not harmed and where benefit to individuals or communities can accrue, research projects should not be rejected by ethics committees purely because there is no written consent. Alternative methods should be explored (subject to Institutional Research Board [IRB]/Research Ethics Committee [REC] or other institutional approval, of course), such as oral consent that is witnessed in written form by a trusted, independent figure, such as a community nurse or religious leader.[1]

Where written consent is possible, but where language barriers preclude the production of the form in the participants' language, local translators should be employed to translate and back-translate the form. Sometimes back-translation is not sufficient and researchers are advised to extensively pilot test their consent forms and procedures for comprehensibility (see Chapter 4). Using local translators can have more than one benefit: accuracy is likely to be enhanced, particularly if dialect-specific or locality-specific terms are necessary, and it is also tangible evidence of local involvement and consultation. The latter point is important in terms of establishing and maintaining trust and credibility.

Local translators can also be used to explore the appropriate comprehension level for the consent process, both oral and written. In addition, they may be aware of subtle meanings of different terms, or may be able to advise on the appropriateness of including or excluding some terms. Some societies, for example, have no words for concepts or objects that Westerners take for granted, such as parasites or diseases, believing instead that illnesses are visited upon them by evil spirits (Crigger *et al.*, 2001). Providing information in an insightful way can help to overcome some of these problems. For example, researchers could refer to an instrument as 'a machine to see how hard your heart is working', as opposed to 'a gauge to measure hydrostatic pressure', or a 'sphygmomanometer' (Crigger *et al.*, 2001). A sport example might be 'a bicycle that doesn't go anywhere', as opposed to a 'cycle ergometer'. It is important, though, to avoid condescension, and this is best achieved through meaningful local consultation when constructing any informed consent process. When considering the informed consent process, researchers should bear in mind that participants may lack education and exposure to scientific concepts. Also, they may not understand the difference between research and health care, and may be confused by the notoriously misunderstood concepts of randomisation and placebos (Dawson and Kass, 2005).

In many societies, those who cannot provide written consent are often marginalised groups or individuals. This may include the diseased, women, the poorly educated or those imprisoned for a variety of reasons, including politics. These categories often comprise the populations who fall under the heading 'vulnerable' as we saw in Chapter 8. A lack of literacy, though, does not preclude participants/subjects from being able to make important decisions about themselves and their communities, but insistence on signed written consent may do so. Thus equity (which we use a shorthand for 'social justice') may become an issue in written informed consent procedures. If ethics committees insist on written consent this may unfairly exclude some members of a community, or whole communities. The injustice entailed can range from exclusion in an exercise and dietary intervention to not receiving the benefits of an advanced trial to test the efficacy of a drug in combating a debilitative disease. In short, insistence on rigid, inappropriate procedures can result in withholding potential benefits from those who need them the most. It can also negatively impact on validity or authenticity by excluding people who have the very characteristics that need to be studied.

Written forms have a different standing according to the value each society places on them. Commonplace in the West, signing a written form may be viewed as an everyday occurrence, perhaps even as an irritation or as something that may provide a limited amount of legal protection. In Egyptian society, however, a signature has particular importance and is usually related to major life events. For example, a signature is most commonly associated with marriage, property, financial and legal matters, rather than a necessary irritation to secure the parcel from the courier at your door. Importantly, being asked to sign a consent form may imply a lack of trust in one's word (consider the response: 'My word is my bond; is that not good enough for you?'). The researcher, asking for a signature may be construed as insulting to the participant if oral consent or assent has already been provided (Rashad *et al.*, 2004).

Detailed written consent can also potentially have a negative effect on participation (and hence validity) in cultures with a more oral tradition. For example, inundating people with information, particularly of a difficult technical nature, may obscure proper understanding of the intentions and implications of a project. This can lead to distrust, which may be exacerbated by a perception that the form is a smokescreen. A form with overly cautious, even exculpatory language, that attempts to excuse the researcher(s) from responsibility, may be viewed something along the lines of 'Methinks they doth protest too much their innocence',[2] and may create suspicion among participants as to the intentions of the researchers. This is of course particularly understandable in Africa, for example, where the conduct of 'outsider' researchers might be construed as echoing previous decades of imperialism.

Culture and values

An awareness of cultural variation and diversity leads to the recognition, and sometimes the adoption too, of different values among and even within societies. Culture, which is learned or inculcated through group interaction, organises human experience and perceptions of experiences. As a dynamic and constantly developing process, culture is shared and is an adaptation to specific environmental and social factors (Barnes *et al.*, 1998).

Despite variations in culture and values, researchers from industrialised countries adopt a Western biomedical approach to medicine- and health-related research, and this powerful force has shaped a dominant and prevailing worldview (Benatar, 2002). The fallout for research ethics is that industrialised nations grant approval to projects that ostensibly satisfy so-called universal ethical standards, often without regard to the values of the populations to be studied (Crigger *et al.*, 2001). As Benatar (2002) has pointed out, however, there is a need to be sensitive (especially with those who are disadvantaged or who have been exploited) and to recognise that they are likely to see the world through different lenses, with different foci and emphasis. Similarly, writing from an Eastern European perspective, Bencko stated that:

> One of the current risks associated with social transition is the tendency to transfer and implant the organisational or legislative principles from 'the West' without any or adequate critical review and adjustment to local Central and Eastern European conditions.
>
> (Bencko, 1996: 80)

Bencko contends that such sudden liberalisation involves some risks, and this view is shared by Crigger *et al.* (2001), who challenge the appropriateness of applying stringent guidelines from individuated countries to some cultures. In support of Bencko, they go so far as to say that the commonly accepted ethics of research may actually do harm by violating values of communities in developing nations. This is of course problematical; non-maleficence (or non-harm) is considered one of the critical components of research ethics in the West, indeed of Western ethics more generally speaking.

The reference to what may be called 'individuated' countries points the way towards one of the difficulties in applying 'Western' standards of research ethics universally. Anglo-American cultural values stress individualism, self-reliance, materialism, technology, independence, achievement and a reliance on the power of science to solve problems (Bellah *et al.*, 1985; Barnes *et al.*, 1998). In contrast, African,[3] central American or Asian cultures tend variously to stress family, communitarian or patriarchal models of decision-making, serving others, deference to elders, compliance with authority, group communal assistance, privacy, the importance of hard work and a reliance on religious or spiritual beliefs and practices.

Western individualism is ethically grounded in the deontological conception of people as ends in themselves. This gives rise to the perceived necessity for informed consent, which applies tenets of rights, autonomy, self-determination and privacy. This, however, is at variance with many non-Western cultures, which stress the embeddings of an individual within society and emphasise relational definitions of personhood (Christakis, 1992).

These differences in values, perceptions and practical decision-making processes can have profound implications for the application of research ethics. In some cultures, for instance, while individual decision-making exists in some forms, there are situations where consent is granted by community or tribal leaders. Or, at the very least, it is expected that such figures be consulted before individuals are approached. A clear requirement for this type of consent though is that the authority figure is acting in good faith on behalf of his or her constituents.[4] This might of course offend Western sensibilities of 'freedom', but it should be recognised that such practices might perform a valuable societal function and that individuals might not necessarily consider themselves 'unfree'. In many African communities, there is a great deal of emphasis placed on family-focused decision-making. It is worth bearing in mind that 'family' here can mean an extended family. This derives from the African cultural notion that one's nieces and nephews are considered to be one's children, and one's aunts and uncles are considered as additional parents. A similar model of deference to family is found in Japan, and these examples illustrate that the 'autonomy-oriented' model of bioethics may not be applicable across individuals and societies (Hipshman, 1999).

Similarly, some cultures practise patriarchal decision-making systems, where the husband, as the head of the household, makes decisions for everyone else. So, in cultures such as these, researchers will find women reluctant to make decisions for themselves or their children without at least consulting their husbands first. Patriarchy can extend to situations where a wife is considered as the husband's property (Dawson and Kass, in press).

In less-developed areas, a substantial proportion of the population may feel that only the father can make decisions about a child's participation in research. However repugnant Western researchers may find this, attempts to impose a universalistic model of research ethics may lead to non-participation in their studies. A culturally sensitive approach will recognise the norms and practices of all societies, and it is important to recognise that this doesn't necessarily mean an acceptance of ethical relativism.

Autonomy is not easily translated into all cultures. Religious or spiritual beliefs also need to be borne in mind when applying processes of research ethics. In Islam, for example, each individual is considered free and answerable only to God. In practice though, in Egyptian society decision-making power is frequently delegated to the most powerful figure in each specific context, such as the father, teacher, employer or doctor. This is further compounded for women by their relative disempowerment in society. Taboos or religious laws might severely restrict participation in studies by some sectors of society. For example, a religious taboo might prevent women being interviewed by strangers (Crosby and Grodin, 2002). Similarly, Islamic holy law (*Sharia*) might prevent skinfold body fat measurement in Muslim women in certain situations, as the measurement will involve various stages of undressing and exposure of the body.

Deference to authority might predispose *towards* participation, resulting in a loss of autonomy for participants. Rashad *et al.* (2004) contend that for Arab women, deference to the medical profession impairs autonomy and the ability to make informed choices about care. In many impoverished societies, health-care professionals or researchers occupy the higher echelons of society and individuals might agree to participate because of unequal power relationships. Leach *et al.* (1999), in a study of informed consent procedures in the Gambia, found that mothers from rural areas admitted that they would have found it difficult to refuse to consent to participation.

Perceived inducement may also play a role in predisposing towards participation. Access to inoculations, for instance, or participation in a weight-reduction programme, could lead participants to consent where they might otherwise not have done so. It is of course laudable that projects might benefit the individuals involved (as well as, hopefully, society at large), but this can be a problem if there is any misunderstanding of potential benefits. In both the health and exercise examples presented above, randomisation, placebos or control groups are likely to apply. These concepts are notoriously misunderstood by populations that have little formal education in the sciences and researchers should be careful to avoid misunderstandings. Not only can personal resentment arise when expected benefits do not accrue, but the distrust created has implications for the conduct of future studies involving those and other disempowered communities.

Of course, this might with some justification be perceived as 'going native' – subscribing uncritically to the norms of the researched. We are not suggesting this. What we are attempting to outline is a research ethic that is context-sensitive. Clearly one cannot change the whole world in and by one's research. There may, however, be cases where one is obliged to gain a patriarchal consent or none, and where one may pursue opportunities to confirm this with those for whom consent – or better 'assent' – has already been granted. In this way we at least in part respect both individual autonomy and the dominant local patterns of authorisation.

Distrust/imperialism

Political and historical factors may create a different kind of distrust where people who are oppressed, or have been oppressed, resent the intrusion of 'outsiders' into their culture, as we saw in Chapter 8, and as captured in the memorable phrase 'nothing about us without us' (Charlton, 1998). In parts of Africa, for example, decades of imperialism and/or colonialism have resulted in a legacy of intense resentment. In these situations, research is viewed historically as something that is done *to* people, even paternalistically *for* people, but not necessarily collaboratively *with* them or *by* them. In this scenario, the research process itself is an expression of the power of the researcher over the researched (French, 1987). Leach *et al.* (1999) found evidence of distrust of the motives of scientists from developed countries working in poorer countries. One participant stated:

these vaccines brought here to Africa by scientists cannot be trusted. Because these Europeans know we are poor people and so accept any terms and conditions, they are using Africans as guinea pigs, and Africa as a dumping place for so much waste.

(Leach *et al.*, 1999: 143)

To explore the issue of mistrust, it might be useful to consider the following fictional narrative[5] which is intended to illustrate the disparities in power between the researchers and the researched:

Sipho is a 52-year-old Zulu male, working as a cane-cutter in rural Zululand. His formal education ended in Grade 2, and he can neither read nor write. He grew up during some of the most miserable years in Apartheid South Africa, where his people were oppressed and denied opportunities and rights such as access to education. His father was killed in fighting between the warring ANC and Inkatha Freedom Party factions in this strife-torn corner of South Africa. His mother died giving birth to her seventh child, Sipho's youngest sister Gugu, who has since died of AIDS. Several of Sipho's friends have died in the same way, in an area where 33 per cent of mothers attending neonatal clinics test positive for HIV.

He lives in a compound with his co-workers and they follow a communal mode of decision-making on matters that affect the group. On Sundays, he travels to the Reserve where his wife and family live. Close family relationships and interdependence are characteristic of his society. His father presides over the extended group in a benign, yet autocratic, way, making decisions for the benefit of the group as a whole. All members of the family contribute to maintaining a reasonable standard of living for the elderly members, as respect for elders is a feature of Zulu culture.

For the equivalent of UK £40 a month, Sipho works eight hours a day cutting sugar cane with a short machete. If he falls ill or injures himself in the dangerous working conditions, he does not get paid for time off and the nearest clinic is a three-hour walk away in the harsh African sun. The compound where he lives with his co-workers belongs to his unsympathetic white boss, who only recently installed a communal tap so that the workers no longer have to collect their water in buckets from the polluted Gwenya river.

Sipho has met white people before, when he was forced to seek work in the city. His time as a gardener in Durban though was miserable, and he felt exploited by the low pay and the disdain in which he was seemingly held by the fast-living, rich, city folk.

Now a group of white researchers, collaborating with the nearby University of Ongoye, want to recruit him to participate in a study. They say that the study is to measure his body's responses to manual labour in hot environments, and that they will capture his breath and take some of his blood.

What are they going to do to his breath? Are they taking his blood because they secretly want to test it for HIV? If they find out that his bodily response is not good, will they tell his boss? If this happens, will his boss replace him with a younger, fitter worker? Who will benefit from this study that they are proposing? What do outsiders know of his working conditions? Are they going to report that he earns next to nothing, and that the food he receives is hardly enough to fill his stomach? Who is going to make the decision about participation, him, the *induna* (foreman), the boss? What will happen to him if he says he doesn't want to take part? Do the researchers care about any of the questions that he has about the study?

The narrative shows the difficulties that researchers from industrialised countries may have in identifying potential problems in transcultural research. 'Have they questioned the extent to which their privileged lives have been constructed and maintained through modern and sophisticated methods of exploitation of people across the globe?' (Benatar, 2002: 1134). Distrust creates a climate where unambiguous exchange of relevant information is impossible and this, in turn, negatively affects a potential participant's ability to make a free and informed choice. Researchers ought to sensitise themselves to issues such as those presented by the narrative, bearing in mind of course that a completely different set of problems may be present in another transcultural setting.

Practical manifestations of distrust can lead to situations where, for example, potential participants give incorrect addresses, thus precluding the possibility of participation or follow up (Leach *et al.*, 1999). Or distrust can result in individual or group refusal to participate. Leach *et al.* (1999) also report an incident where all the mothers in a village refused to join an inoculation trial, and this was communicated through a respected, elderly woman, who stated that 'All the mothers and fathers including the village chief do not want MRC and we have agreed that nobody should accept your interview.' This example illustrates the combination both of mistrust, and of communal decision-making that is uncommon in Westernised countries.

Mistrust can be exacerbated by the consent process itself, paradoxically, by the constant assurance of anonymity, for example, creating an atmosphere of suspicion. Particularly in authoritarian cultures, being offered a choice may seem suspicious. Moreover, in the absence of external verification, rumours can have an adverse effect on building collaborative research relationships.

Between universality and relativism

Some of the difficulties of applying conventional models of research in cultural contexts have been outlined above. These problems are the practical manifestation of tension between applying universal norms (also referred to as moral fundamentalism) or accepting ethical relativism (often implied in the term 'multiculturalism'). So far in this chapter we have seen that, despite the recent emphasis on Western models of bioethics, there is still much debate on whether ethical principles are common across cultures and can therefore be universally applied, or whether they are relative to each culture and must be applied individually (Barnes *et al.*, 1998).

Universality holds that the principles we adopt and translate into processes are fundamental, and ought to be applied to all research settings, across countries and cultures. This is of course the position adopted by the industrialised nations following Nuremberg, and is articulated in the proposal and profusion of binding regulatory systems. The idea of universality in research ethics principles is appealing for a number of reasons. First, the universal systems advocated, being based on the principles of beneficence, justice, non-maleficence and respect for autonomous persons, are intuitively morally attractive. Second, being primarily deontological in nature, their codifications make it relatively easy for practitioners or ethics committees to apply the systems, as extensive moral deliberation is rendered obsolete through prescribed courses of action (e.g. you must obtain first-person informed consent). Third, as the doctrine of industrialised nations, the growth of universal ethics systems is congruent with globalisation in other areas. It is easier, after all, to apply the views of the culturally dominant.

Given that ethical guidelines are generally based on profound religious and philosophical beliefs which may differ across cultures and countries, it follows that ethics regarding research might, *a priori*, be expected to vary across cultures. Conflict is thus likely to emerge where there is direct contact between potentially different systems, where the researcher and the researched come from different cultural backgrounds (Christakis, 1992). The contention that, since ethics are socially constructed, they will vary cross-culturally, is known as relativism. As we saw in Chapter 2, relativism 'appreciates alternative choices and actions' (Crigger *et al.*, 2001: 462), and takes explicit cognisance of context and culture. This is itself intuitively morally attractive, but just as we cautioned against accepting a relativist approach to ethics generally, so too we reject a relativistic research ethics. While we recognise the inherent inflexibility of universalist approaches, we reject the relativist notion that one opinion is equally as good or bad as another. This pandering equates to the very collapse of ethics itself.

While researchers and ethics committees should carefully consider context and cultural values, it does not necessarily follow that what it is right to do or good to be depends simply on the culture to which one belongs. This leads us to accept that there are certain authoritative moral imperatives (such as beneficence, justice and respect for persons), and that these can be applied through a consideration of culture and context despite their Western heritage. In this way we do not fall foul of the genetic fallacy: the logician's warning that a given (say) policy, prescription or proscription is right or wrong simply in virtue of where it emanates from. For example, informed consent is a process, not a principle or a value. As a process, it is based on an acknowledgment of the principle of respect for persons. The principle can still be adhered to, without necessarily following a mechanistic, inflexible process that may alienate and even disempower individuals. Informed consent is about providing adequate, relevant information in a manner and setting that enables someone to make a choice about participation. Providing such information through alternative means, such as video, focus groups, facilitatory discussions with recognised cultural leaders, and so on, can retain the integrity of the process while at the same time showing respect for local values and traditions.

Crigger *et al.* (2001) contend that a culturally sensitive application of research ethics accepts limitations (such as barriers to understanding scientific concepts) as a cultural phenomenon. They argue that investigators should proceed with such projects on the basis of a favourable utilitarian outcome. For example, a rural study that involves health screening may have beneficial outcomes for society at large and for participants, with little or no risk to the individual.[6] While this might seem attractive, the utilitarian nature of the decision-making should not blind researchers to considering the rights of participants.

Let us take an example. One reason for this is that African societies are changing fairly rapidly, through the influence of globalisation in many fields, in ways that make informed consent requirements more rather than less appropriate. Besides, understanding of the research process ultimately happens at an individual level (Dawson and Kass, in press), and this is a further reason for retaining the core aspects of the current Western bioethics model. Supporting this, Ijsellmuiden and Faden contend that:

> The most fundamental argument against modifying the obligation of researchers to obtain informed consent from individual subjects is that such an obligation expresses important and basic moral values that are universally applicable, regardless of variations in cultural practice.
>
> (Ijsellmuiden and Faden, 1992: 830)

This view holds that the principle of respect for persons is inviolable, and the implication of accepting this is that participants have a basic right to choose whether or not to participate, having been given sufficient information to make a free decision. This is of course not to say that consent must be written, or that cultural factors such as communitarian models of decision-making should be ignored. But, 'The assumption that adults in developing countries are mentally incompetent to give informed consent to participation in research is false, if not downright insulting' (Ijsellmuiden and Faden, 1992: 832). To naïvely insist on, for example, a paternalistic approach, or to justify a decision on utilitarian grounds, is to disrespect the participants and their society. The challenge for researchers is to create a process that accords with local customs and values while enabling individuals to make a choice. There are no easy answers here, nor fault-free principles to be deductively applied.

How, then, can respect be shown in practice, when we have seemingly irreconcilable approaches to decision-making, or when there is no shared understanding of health, illness or scientific concepts? Extra efforts are needed to communicate with participants in transcultural contexts. This might mean that questions of justice and freedom, however divisive they might be, should be introduced into debates about the aims and conduct of the research, and should have a bearing on every project (French, 1987). To insist that cultural differences preclude understanding might be, at worst, insulting and disrespectful or might be indicative of a lack of effort on behalf of investigators. As Ijsellmuiden and Faden have said, 'cultural differences do not constitute insurmountable barriers to obtaining valid consent or refusal' (1992: 832). We should be culturally sensitive. We should avoid ethnocentricity. We should appreciate other cultures and their values. Yet, careful ethical analysis should be the background for our decisions on research ethics, and we should make decisions on the basis of acceptance of the principles of beneficence, justice and respect for persons.

Regulatory systems

The regulation of research and mechanisms of ethical approval have been discussed in Chapter 3 and we will not re-examine the general issues in detail here. Nevertheless, transcultural research poses some questions for systems of governance and these are mentioned here. Is ethical approval of both governing systems required? What are researchers to do if regulations conflict? If only one avenue of approval is possible (for example if no regulation exists in a developing country) is that sufficient? These are valid questions, particularly given that the increasing domination of Western conceptions of research ethics is being accompanied by a concomitant rise in transcultural research. To what extent can we apply universalistic notions in order to avoid the capriciousness that relativism can give rise to? Given our previous assertions about the value of very general ethical considerations, it would be inconsistent for us to suggest any sort of relativist mechanisms for ethical regulation. Nevertheless, we recognise that the commonly accepted Western notions of bioethics may be inflexible and inappropriate in some areas of transcultural research.

Of course, in some situations, researchers are bound by regulations set by the systems whereby they obtained original ethical approval. This may prove problematic as such regulations can be impractical in developing countries. IRBs or RECs need to be sensitised to issues in transcultural research, and grant proposers or project directors should, in the early stages of project design and submission, identify potential problems and solutions. In addition, they should write into their projects the necessity and mechanisms for ongoing ethical referral and approval, as research in transcultural projects may pose unanticipated ethical problems that need a swift resolution if the aims of the project are to be realised. Researchers should not only anticipate problems, but they should also attempt to sensitise ethics committees to the issues, by including potential problems and ethically acceptable solutions in their proposals.

Context sensitive research ethics: a case study

How can we make the sorts of decisions about processes that we have alluded to in previous sections, particularly in transcultural situations? Let us return again to the narrative of Sipho, and see what the group of researchers might do to allay his concerns.

Alastair and Luke are ergonomists from the University of Berwick upon Tweed. The former speaks with a broad Scottish accent that most Englishmen struggle to get to grips with, while the latter is young, and aggressively confident in the power of science to solve problems. Their collective social conscience led them to apply for, and receive, a generous grant to quantify the physical demands of manual labour in hot conditions, with the aim of improving efficiency and production. Having well-developed social consciences, they also intend to suggest improvements in working practices, such as introducing frequent hydration breaks for the workers, if this will improve efficiency.

Fortunately, they have reflected on and recognised the potential difficulties that their language, backgrounds and beliefs might pose for their study. Their initial approach to the University of Ongoye was facilitated by a colleague who had previously visited there. Unable to hold a videoconference due to the lack of facilities at Ongoye, they engaged in protracted email and telephone conversations with the researcher at that end, Sabelo Mkhize, and his head of department. They agreed to employ Sabelo as their research assistant if their grant application was successful.

For pilot testing they would use students from Ongoye and they proposed to pay them for their participation. This was deemed problematic, however, as there was no history of paying subjects for participation at the university, and setting a precedent would compromise voluntary participation in future departmental studies, as virtually all research conducted there was unfunded. They settled on a compromise with the head of department – they would make a donation to the Sports Science Students Society, with the monies intended for the educational benefit of students.

Before drafting an interview schedule, Sabelo, armed with letters from the University of Berwick upon Tweed, met with the farm owner, with the headman of the compound, and with the *induna* (foreman). He explained the purpose of the study, the operational processes, the benefits for efficiency and working conditions, and the operational processes, including obtaining consent. He sought consent to proceed from the farmer, then the headman and then the *induna*, in that order, as dictated by the hierarchical structure of the group. He stressed that free and voluntary participation was important for the validity of the study and explained that group consent was unlikely to achieve this. To illustrate the importance of this, he explained that, for example, if people felt coerced or deceived in any way, then they might modify their work patterns (e.g. not work as hard as normal, or work harder) in order to achieve whatever agenda they set for themselves from the study. One way to negate this was to fully inform the participants as to the aims, importance and methods of the study and to allow them to freely choose whether to participate. Sabelo received permission to approach individuals.

Concurrently, Alastair, as project leader, had convinced the local research ethics committee that written informed consent could not be achieved in all cases. Consent procedures would be as follows: a community meeting, convened by the headman and attended by the *induna*, would inform the entire group of the study. They would be told that they would be approached by Sabelo, who would ask them to participate. They were free to decline, with no sanction whatsoever being imposed. They would be paid at a rate equivalent to that normally paid by the University of Berwick upon Tweed. Alastair and Luke recognised that this sum, when converted into the local currency, might constitute undue coercion, as it represented a week's wages in local terms, but felt that to withhold any of this money would be disrespectful to the participants and would devalue their effort relative to participants elsewhere.

The information sheet and consent form had been translated into isiZulu, adjusted for linguistic appropriateness, and back-translated into English. Where necessary, adjustments were made to eliminate technical terms, and it was again translated and back-translated as a final check. Where participants were literate, they would read and sign the form, after a cooling-off period of one week. The cooling-off period was specifically included to give potential participants time to reflect and to allow them to consult with others, such as family members or co-workers. Where they were not literate, oral information was given in the presence of a local nurse who had also been employed using funds from the grant, and participants were invited to give oral consent in a week's time, such consent again being witnessed by the nurse, who attested to this in writing.

Particular efforts were made to stress the independence of the project. Sabelo had to explain that the farmer and headman had been approached first as a matter of courtesy, and that individuals were free to choose whether to participate. Explanations were difficult as several participants felt that to not participate might be perceived as a sign of dissidence. The only way to overcome this was to stress the anonymity of results and data storage. The suspicion of data misuse was particularly strong. How could the researchers convince potential participants that their data would not, for example, be used for promotion/demotion, or that their blood would not be tested for HIV?

Eventually, Alastair and Luke decided to run a mock pilot test/ demonstration for potential participants. With the nurse present to explain what the data meant, the researchers volunteered themselves for a trial. They demonstrated the assignation of code names rather than actual names, showed how identifiers would be kept separate from any actual data, and got the farmer, headman and *induna* to attest that they would not have access to any of the results. The nurse explained what the blood tests would be used for and confirmed the disposal methods, to ensure that no latent tests could be conducted.

The potential broader benefits were confirmed and participants were assured that they could withdraw at any time, with no loss of benefits (that is, they could retain their participation fee if they withdrew). They were given the opportunity to ask questions both in the group setting and during their individual consent procedures. The participant group was also invited to nominate one of their members as a contact person to relay confidential questions or problems to Sabelo, and were assured that they could also approach him individually if they so wished. The potential participant group was also told that the anonymous results of the study would be discussed with them as a group, once analysis had been completed. They would have a chance to provide input into the findings and implications and these would be incorporated into the reports relayed to the Zululand Rural Development Trust, to the Kwazulu Health and Safety Board, to the University of Ongoye and to the funding body.

The ideal outcome of the fictional situation described above would be that participants understood the relevant implications, that they volunteered, and that the successfully published and widely acclaimed study resulted in significant improvements to both efficiency and working conditions of cane-cutters. However, the actions described above would probably not be as clear-cut or as easily applied as the narrative suggests. Suspicion about the motives for and the use of data might remain, and the decision-making process, including the involvement of the farmer and the *induna*, might prove problematic. Also, the payment might be construed as offering undue inducement. Nevertheless, we do not think it is defeatist to recognise that not all problems can be solved. In making decisions about the effect of procedures on ethics, we want to do the best that we can in the circumstances. This is of course assuming that the results of the study are important, that participants benefit or are not harmed, and that their rights are preserved.

Conclusion

Transcultural research poses particular problems, and it is incumbent on researchers to identify these, reflect on them, and propose culturally sensitive and context-sensitive solutions. The challenges for researchers are to avoid both ethical imperialism and relativism, to design studies that are valid and authentic, to contribute to the development of communities with which they collaborate, and to respect group and individual rights. A step towards implementing this might be to recognise that 'Being respectful of individuals requires attention to the context in which individuals and families live and make decisions' (Dawson and Kass, in press). Transculturalism presents us with some tricky ethical difficulties, but the difficulty in achieving dialogue doesn't mean that efforts should be abandoned. As Christakis has argued, 'We must navigate, in short, between the simplicity of ethical universality and the evasion and complexity of ethical relativism, between intellectual hubris and moral paralysis' (1992: 1089).

10 Research and society
Is bad science *ipso facto* bad ethics?

What are the ethical limits to research? We saw in Chapter 1 how sometimes good motives brought about ethically indefensible research and we questioned whether good use might be made of morally culpable research. These are some of the easier questions when examining more globally the relationship between research and ethics. A subtle problem, confronted frequently by Institutional Research Boards (IRBs) and Research Ethics Committees (RECs), concerns the matter of how one can precisely draw lines between the ethical dimensions of research and the epistemological or methodological ones. And this is no easy matter. How should we think about gene therapy to combat muscular dystrophy or Erythropoietin (EPO) for circulation difficulties, which is then used to assist violations of commonly accepted sports rules? What about research into psychological preparation which is used to motivate players to such an extent that they knowingly injure other athletes? Or what if we study the ergonomic implications of holding a shooting rifle in a certain position for biathlon competitors, with obvious potential consequences for future harm beyond sports? These simple examples raise deep questions about ethics and research. Some are more direct in their implications than others. While it has been suggested that the ethical review of research should (somehow) cauterise the epistemological from the ethical, it is not always possible and sometimes it is not desirable to do this. What we shall aim to achieve in this final chapter is a consideration of the reasonable limits researchers and IRBs/RECs might consider in the development and appraisal of research projects.

The research/ethics duplex in research governance

If one talks to members of IRBs/RECs about why they spend so much time discussing the scientific design of a project, you are likely to get a response along the lines that they have to be sure that the science is good because 'Bad research (or, more often, bad science) equals bad ethics.' For many people it is a *sine qua non* of research ethics that to be ethically acceptable a project must be of sound scientific research design. Is this necessarily the case?

One of the key sets of international guidelines on research ethics, from the Council for International Organizations of Medical Sciences (CIOMS), makes it clear in its guidelines that it considers bad science to be ethically indefensible:

> *Guideline 1: Ethical justification and scientific validity of biomedical research involving human beings*
>
> The ethical justification of biomedical research involving human subjects is the prospect of discovering new ways of benefiting people's health. Such research can be ethically justifiable only if it is carried out in ways that respect and protect, and are fair to, the subjects of that research and are morally acceptable within the communities in which the research is carried out. Moreover, *because scientifically invalid research is unethical* in that it exposes research subjects to risks without possible benefit, investigators and sponsors must ensure that proposed studies involving human subjects conform to generally accepted scientific principles and are based on adequate knowledge of the pertinent scientific literature.
>
> (CIOMS, 2002, emphasis added)

The document goes on to elaborate this principle in some detail, arguing that an 'essential feature' of ethical research is that 'the research offers a means of developing information not otherwise obtainable, that the design of the research is scientifically sound, and that the investigators and other research personnel are competent' and that 'Investigators and sponsors must also ensure that all who participate in the conduct of the research are qualified by virtue of their education and experience to perform competently in their roles' (CIOMS, 2002).

At first sight, these strictures seem uncontroversial. Surely we would not wish to involve people in taking part in research, at some personal inconvenience and possibly risk of harm, if the project were so ill-conceived that there was little or no prospect of benefit from the research. Does accepting the notion that research should be beneficent not require this? Should members of IRBs/RECs, in carrying out their roles, prevent research participants from being exposed to incompetent researchers? We will argue that the problem is often not quite so straightforward as it might unthinkingly seem. In this chapter we will analyse the claim that 'bad science equals bad ethics' and suggest that, at the very least, we need a more subtle account than is usually offered.

The CIOMS guidelines are particularly aimed at medical research – including sports medicine[1] – though their reach might well be thought to extend into the overlaps with exercise and health sciences. The scope and variety of sports sciences – traditionally thought of as sports biomechanics, sports physiology and sports psychology but here used in the broader European sense to refer to any disciplined research – extends beyond the confines of biomedical science.[2] However, there is a lack of comparable international guidelines for exercise and sports science research ethics, and we would argue that the relationship between sports and exercise science and health or medical science is so close as to make the CIOMS and similar research ethics guidance relevant and worthy of critical reflection. Of course, not all exercise and sports sciences research is aimed at performance enhancement. To the contrary, a substantial proportion – perhaps even the majority – is intimately connected with the health and well-being of broader populations, with the objectives of reducing risk of injury, improving treatments, creating safer training environments and demonstrating the mental, physical and societal benefits that are connected with exercise.

Participants in such research may be subjected to exceptionally physically demanding procedures at no small cost, physically, to themselves and potentially at some personal risk. The results of such work will be generalised to the wider population and taken up by a range of people in different settings. Therefore, any interventions or recommendations as to exercise or training regimes, as with medical treatments, must be rigorously tested. If we transfer these ideas into the CIOMS guidelines, we might say that the ethical justification of research in exercise and sport sciences is that it holds out the prospect of improving fitness, or health and well-being, or enhancing physical performance or the quality of participation in a variety of physically active pursuits. Even if this were to be reduced to aims such as improving health, albeit in a narrow and particular conception of health (as species-typical functioning)[3] and improving performance the argument we offer will apply. Research involving human subjects in the name of exercise and sports sciences that offered no prospect of such benefit might thus be thought to be unethical. Of course, research that improved performance of some, perhaps at the expense of the participants, or other performers' health, would also be unethical.

Are there essential features of ethical research?

Ethical merit in research at the very least embraces respect for the dignity of participants. As we have argued throughout the book, this includes, among other things, safeguarding their privacy, ensuring their safety and acknowledging their human rights. It also involves obligations on the part of researchers to assess and minimise risk, to perform risk–benefit assessments, to avoid conflicts of interest, to provide recompense or reward where appropriate, to provide compensation for injury and to preserve anonymity and confidentiality where appropriate.[4]

Before moving to the central features of our argument, it might be worth, as an aside, introducing the notion of consideration of future consequences raised in Chapter 2, in our critical remarks on consequentialist ethical theories. How far ought we to go in trying to determine the potential impact of our research? For example, imagine that you are a sports scientist with particular expertise in ergonomics. As part of a much larger-scale project, you might be asked to do some contract research to determine optimal comfort and alertness relating to a seated position in a cramped space. The aim is to design a seat that is both comfortable and functional, with the best characteristics to ensure visual recognition and associated manually dextrous activity. It might be easy to conceive of such research being sponsored by a Formula 1 racing team. Imagine, by contrast, that the sponsor is a military department of the government and you have been asked to design a seat inside a battle tank, where the operator will sight, aim and fire on selected (lawful?) targets.

At first glance, your research does not seem to contravene any of the principles outlined above (Benatar, 2002), not least because your participants will not suffer any harms while engaging in your research. Your research may in fact be methodologically rigorous; it may follow sound tenets of data collection, but is it ethically defensible? Clearly, research of this nature carries the potential to contribute significantly to harming others. You, as the researcher, are obliged to consider the future consequences of your work. Does this mean that we should attempt to suppress advances in science that could be used for harmful ends (as well as good ones)? Of course not. Yet it does introduce the notion that we should consider, to some extent, how we manage science for the greater good, rather than just engaging with the technical procedures of science.

More specifically, for the purposes of our argument, according to the most recent CIOMS guidelines, the essential features of ethically justified research involving human subjects could be paraphrased for exercise, health and sports and sciences as follows:

- The research must offer the prospect of discovering new ways of benefiting people's health, well-being, fitness or performance, or improving the quality of their participation in physical activities.
- The research must offer a means of developing information not otherwise obtainable.
- The research must conform to generally accepted scientific principles and be based on adequate knowledge of the pertinent scientific literatures.
- The investigators and other research personnel must be competent.
- The methods to be used must be appropriate to the objectives of the research and the field of study.
- The research must be carried out in ways that respect, protect and are fair to the subjects of that research, and that are acceptable within the communities in which the research is carried out.[5]

Put more formally, an argument can be constructed which runs roughly as follows:

1   The ethical justification for research is the prospect of discovering ways of benefiting health, fitness, participation, etc.

2   The information sought cannot be obtained by other means.
3   Only research that respects, protects and is fair to the research subjects is ethically acceptable.
4   Research exposes subjects to risks.
5   A (proportionate) degree of risk can be accepted if there are expected benefits (i.e. benefit in better ways of achieving health and fitness or promoting participation etc.).
6   Scientifically invalid research offers no prospect of (these kinds of) benefits.

Therefore:

7   Scientifically invalid research is unethical.

Do these essential features of research amount to a valid argument?

Premise 1 states that the ethical justification for research is the prospect of discovering new ways to benefit people's fitness, well-being, etc. through the creation of generalisable new knowledge. Everything else that follows in the argument takes this as its starting point and we might well be prepared to accept it as true. But is this type of benefit the only (or supreme) ethical justification, or just one among others (notwithstanding its importance)? If we are to agree with the conclusion of the argument, we have to accept that it is the only justification, but this is never explicitly stated. The assumption seems to be that the only ethically significant benefit is the scientific benefit of obtaining new knowledge that cannot be obtained in any other way, and no account can be taken of other possible benefits, for example to the participant, the researcher or society. What if there were other plausible ethical justifications apart from the prospect of narrowly defined scientific benefit? Indeed, should research whose effects are neither significantly harmful nor beneficial other than as an educational tool be rejected by IRBs or RECs?

One situation alluded to in Chapter 2, in which RECs[6] frequently come up against complaints that a project cannot possibly generate new knowledge is that of the student project. Many students on undergraduate and graduate programmes are expected to produce a dissertation and this is frequently based on a piece of empirical research. In some subjects it may be possible to conduct such projects in the laboratory or the library, using sources of data other than living human subjects. In the UK at least, certain university departments have simply stopped undergraduates gaining empirical data where this has required Local Research Ethics Committee (LREC) approval for this, and also for reasons of time and expediency. But in disciplines such as psychology, the social sciences, health sciences and sports and exercise science, students not unreasonably desire to carry out projects using human participants. For many students, of course, the constraints of time-scales, other courses or modules, financial resources and so on will mean their projects must necessarily be small scale. This in turn will limit their scientific merit, as will their status as novice researchers – after all, the purpose of the project is for the student to learn about research. If we accept the dictum that 'bad science equals bad ethics', these projects will therefore be unethical. This is surely an inappropriate application of the principle.

A fictional example may assist in teasing out just some of the issues. Imagine you are a sports sciences lecturer who has been assigned a total of 13 undergraduate dissertation projects to supervise (a scandalous but not infrequent allocation). One of these deals with attitudes towards structured versus unstructured physical activity, using children as research subjects. Using a semantic differential attitude scale as the data collection instrument, your student has the laudable aim of making recommendations as to which mode of activity best serves to motivate children with regard to participation in physical activity. In the analysis section of the research proposal, she suggests that she will treat the data as interval, for purposes of comparative statistical analysis.

Given your workload of 13 students, and given that this is not a specialist area of yours, you do what reading you are able to and agree to supervise the research as proposed by the student. In your university, all studies using human subjects/participants must pass ethical scrutiny, in this case the departmental ethics sub-committee comprising the normal range of members (see Chapter 3). One of the members (perhaps an external member, who may be unfamiliar with the methods of your discipline), takes issue with the fact that the data are considered interval rather than, say ordinal. The member (probably incorrectly) suggests that the suggested related t-test is inappropriate, and the project is referred back to the student for revision.

There are several issues to consider here. First, should an ethics committee concern itself with matters that are not overtly ethical *per se*, such as statistical applications? Put differently, even if the committee member were correct in his interpretation, should they raise the issue at all? Perhaps we might resolve that the reservations should only turn into recommendations if there are ethically significant repercussions arising from the 'bad' statistics.[7] If the project were to go ahead as proposed (and even assuming that the proposed analysis were incorrect), it is difficult to see what harm might result. Of course, it could be argued that there is always harm to subjects, however insignificant it might be, such as occupying time that might have been more profitably used. What though, of the goods produced? In this case, the subjects/participants may have enjoyed participation, and it may have led them to think more deeply about their enjoyment of physical activity. Also, and importantly, we need to recognise that no project is perfect, and there is an educational benefit to researchers inherent in all research. In this case the student would benefit through the assessment process, and in more sophisticated work researchers benefit through both collaboration with peers and through scrutiny of proposals and of work intended for publication.

A second issue relates to the statement above that no work is perfect. Does the failure to attain a (mythical) 'gold standard' mean that no attempt should be made? Perhaps an analogy may be helpful here. The same student, deemed statistically inept by the research ethics reviewer, also has the misfortune to be a particularly poor amateur (Sunday league) soccer player. Nevertheless, she happily and enthusiastically turns out for every practice and game that her team is involved in. She enjoys both the social interaction and the health benefits that arise from this, and, in addition, her standard of play marginally improves. There are benefits both to her and her team-mates arising from her non-expert participation. Would we want to exclude her from participation because she is not good enough to play in a higher division? Similarly, would we want to prevent her conducting the research because her knowledge of inferential statistics is deemed inadequate? Bear in mind that in both cases judgement is being delivered by someone who is not necessarily an expert – a team selector on the one hand and an external committee member on the other.

Of course ethical review is rarely as simple as these scenarios might imply. If she were a poor enough player so as to constitute a danger to others, for example through overenthusiastic but technically dangerous tackling, then her team might want to coach her appropriately until she has the requisite skills. Similarly, if the conduct of her research were to have negative consequences for participants, then the project ought to be rejected, with specific advice for improvements. Also, one area of poorly designed projects that does have an ethical implication is that of misuse, even unintentionally, of resources. So if resources were to be allocated to a project (including funding and staff time), then poor design or analysis becomes an issue. Nevertheless, this is unlikely in a student project. It is our contention that, whether in football or research, we learn by our mistakes. It may be that in some cases 'bad' science equals 'bad' ethics, but this is not always necessarily so, particularly if harms are difficult to identify and if there are probable educational benefits.

The key question here is the purpose of student projects and the benefits expected from them. The objectives of most higher education programmes are to introduce students to new ideas and information and to develop intellectual skills and abilities. Typically the latter would include the ability to think critically and analytically, to speculate about ideas and questions and to be able to understand how one's speculations and questions might be answered. Where students' questions or hypotheses are of the type that can be answered by empirical inquiry an important part of the student's intellectual development is the ability to work out what information would be required to provide an answer, what would count as evidence for or against an hypothesis, how such evidence might be gathered and analysed and so on. These of course are transferable skills: anyone who has been trained in the methods of empirical inquiry will be able to apply the same logic and systematic approach to problem-solving in other settings. They will also be more likely to examine the claims of others in a critical fashion, knowing how to read a research report and having insight into the process of question formulation, research design, methods of analysis and what is or is not a reasonable conclusion to be drawn from a given data set.

Such skills are important general life skills and contribute something to the employability of graduates, so in a very general way the skills of research contribute to the general public good that comes from higher education. We are constantly reminded of the importance of graduates to the health of the economy and the general good of society, and to some extent that good depends on students receiving training in the skills of systematic inquiry. More specifically, many undergraduate and postgraduate qualifications these days have a strong vocational element, providing qualifications in the professions, such as education, health care, social services and so on. If we leave aside debates about the true value of the professions for society[8] and simply acknowledge the extent to which society is dependent upon the professions in almost every aspect of life, the education and training of the professions, and particularly those involved in public services and what might be called the helping professions, we can see that the proper education of such people makes a significant contribution to the greater good. We all want our doctors, nurses, physiotherapists, teachers, trainers and coaches to provide the best possible service, and that in part depends on the quality of the education they receive. This education includes making mistakes under supervised conditions and learning from them. In particular, professionals who intervene in our lives in significant ways, with the potential to do us great harm if they pursue the wrong intervention, must be able critically to assess the evidence on which they base their practice. That is why we trust them.

Of course, some of our students will go on themselves to become academics and researchers. The beginnings of such future careers may well have their roots in that first experience of the independent, self-directed study provided by the final year project or the Master's degree dissertation. If we accept the need for such people and believe that they contribute something worthwhile to society then again we must accept the possibility of a benefit. Our proposition is thus that the prospect of a project generating new knowledge, of a level and quality that will significantly change practice for example, while an important and morally relevant benefit of research, is not the only such benefit. If we accept that student projects (with their inevitable mistakes and the attendant educational gains) contribute something useful to the education of the student, then that may also be a morally relevant benefit. One ethical test for a student project thus becomes: is it educationally sound and will it contribute in some way to an educational benefit? It is important to note that these questions do not replace those concerning the ends and means of the research to achieve their desired goal. They simply supplant an overly zealous scientific demand for originality and beneficial consequences beyond that which is reasonable.

The second premise in the argument is that the information to be gained from the research cannot be obtained by other means and this is also a sound principle in research generally. However, if we accept that the primary objective of the student project is educational rather than scientific we can rephrase this to say that the expected educational benefit cannot be obtained by other means. We will leave it to the designers of curricula and the educational researchers to tackle this problem in depth, but it seems reasonable to suggest that, while the process of data analysis for example could be learned through work on dummy data sets or secondary analysis, it would be difficult to replicate the experience of organising data collection and actually conducting the interviews or carrying out the tests required to generate the data through simulation exercises.

The third premise refers to the requirement in the CIOMS guidelines that only research that respects and protects the participants is ethically acceptable. The notion of respect here can be seen as fulfilling the Kantian injunction to treat people always as ends in themselves and never merely as means to an end. Clearly we all use others to help us achieve our ends and similarly we allow others to use us, but this is normally within some structure of acknowledgement and consent. It is the asking permission and the acceptance of the autonomy of the other and his or her right to refuse that provides the respect for the other as an end in him or herself. In our everyday leisure and work lives we frequently take this for granted, with consent most often being implied or assumed. Nevertheless, it is noteworthy that when we feel someone has overstepped the mark, either socially or in the context of employment, we are inclined to take offence and complain about being taken for granted.

Respect and risks, protection and privacy

The protection of the research participant is a key element of research ethics. As we have mentioned elsewhere, all research involving human participants involves some kind of cost to the participant. This may be trivial, involving no more than the agreement that some piece of information, collected in the course of routine practice, may be used as data in some research. If, for example, a sports therapist has treated a series of clients with a particular kind of injury and recorded measurements of the clients' progress, she might wish to collect this data together, analyse the effectiveness of certain treatments in certain types of case and publish the results. If she seeks the permission of the clients to use this data, already collected in the course of the treatment, the cost to the client is minimal but, nevertheless, does exist.

If, on the other hand, the research is into some aspect of respiratory physiology or cardiovascular function, for example, requiring participants to attend the laboratory for lengthy periods, undertake strenuous exercise on an ergometer to the point of exhaustion and give blood, urine or other specimens, the cost is considerable in terms of the time taken, the attendant opportunity costs and the pain and discomfort involved. There may even be some degree of physical risk: it is not for nothing that when treadmill tests are performed on cardiac patients in the health setting it is at least desirable – and perhaps ought to be obligatory – that someone in attendance is trained in emergency first aid and advanced life-support procedures.

It is thus incumbent on researchers to make sure that the risk or cost to the participant is minimised and is in keeping with the objectives of the research. The history of research has many examples of researchers taking what seem now to be grave risks, often with their own lives and sometimes with others. For example, in the development of anaesthetics, nitrous oxide (Sir Humphrey Davy) and chloroform (James Simpson) were tried out by the doctors who first thought of using them. Curare, however, was first used as a muscle relaxant by Howard Randal Griffiths on 23 January 1942 in a patient undergoing appendicectomy. Wynands (1998: n.p.) remarks: 'He understood the problems with curare and while others would try it in a laboratory and abandon it, he with wisdom and courage used it in the operating room and demonstrated it to be safe', an attitude that a modern ethics committee might find difficult to accept.

These days it is generally thought to be the role of IRBs/RECs to review research proposals and to make judgements about questions of risk and benefit. Savulescu has argued, for example, that: 'The first responsibility of ethics committees should be to ensure that the expected harm associated with participation is reasonable' (2001: 148) and he goes on to claim that: 'It is a mistake to give more weight to consent than to expected harm. Ethics committees must make an evaluation of the expected harm and whether less harmful avenues should be pursued' (2001: 150). However, this position has its critics. For some people, in acting in this way the research ethics committee is taking an unduly paternalistic stance. Edwards *et al.* (2004) argue that 'research ethics committees (RECs) should not be paternalistic by rejecting research that poses risk to people competent to decide for themselves' (2004: 88) and that 'RECs should not be more restrictive than the "normal" constraints on people taking risks with themselves' (2004: 88).

Both Savulescu and Edwards *et al.* (2004) base their respective arguments, noted briefly in Chapter 4, upon some very difficult examples; the deaths of Jesse Gelsinger and Ellen Roche. Gelsinger was an 18-year-old man who suffered from a mild form of an inherited metabolic disorder which, in his case, could be well controlled with diet and medication. He volunteered to take part in the early trials of gene therapy for the condition, apparently with the altruistic desire to help others, including infants who had the more severe, fatal form of the condition; there was no prospect of benefit for him from his participation. Roche was a healthy volunteer who took part in a study of respiratory function that involved her inhaling a substance that would induce an asthma-like reaction, constricting her airways. In both cases the researchers and those who approved the studies would argue that the participants were given full information about the study and the attendant risks and were competent to make an informed decision. This is particularly relevant in the case of Gelsinger, as it was decided to use adults with the mild form of the condition rather than infants with the inevitably fatal form, as the former could give a competent consent where the latter could not; it is generally accepted that incompetent individuals should only be recruited to research involving minimal harm.

What, if anything, can such dramatic examples tell us about more mundane student projects? First, they remind us that even in studies involving healthy volunteers and procedures that in most cases would cause no harm, unexpected tragedies can occur. Gelsinger, for example, was the eighteenth and last patient in the trial and none of the other participants were affected. Second, they suggest that there should be a very tough limit on the kind of research that students should be allowed to conduct. This is one area where minimal harm really must be assured. Savulescu goes on to suggest that:

> it is important to distinguish between the *chance* of a bad outcome occurring and *expected harm*. Expected harm is the probability of a harm occurring multiplied by the magnitude of that harm. Being harmed by an intervention is being made worse off than one would otherwise have been if that intervention had not been performed.
>
> (Savulescu, 2001: 149)

If we accept Savulescu's position over the more relaxed position of Edwards *et al.*, it would still seem permissible to allow participants the opportunity to take part in a student project that involved them in, say, mild inconvenience or some degree of stress. There is, of course, always going to be the chance of harm. The participant might be involved in a traffic accident on the way to take part in the research, a journey he would not otherwise have undertaken. An athlete accustomed to hard training might nevertheless experience a cardiac event while on the research ergometer test but, given that he trained in this way on a regular basis, this would seem to be chance harm rather than an expected harm. But both the chance of harm and any harm that could possibly be expected must be minimised if the accompanying benefit is educational rather than scientific.

What, to use the words of Edwards *et al.* (2004), would constitute 'the "normal" constraints on people taking risks with themselves'? One analogy that might be useful is that of product liability. Current legislation imposes strict liability on producers or manufacturers for harm caused by defective products. This creates an important distinction between risks I might take with myself and risks to which others may expose me. So, if I wish to take up rock climbing and make myself a harness out of a couple of old belts stitched together, the risk I take is my own and if the harness breaks the first time I try to abseil with it, the fault is mine. If I purchase a climbing harness from a manufacturer and the first time I use it, it breaks because the materials were shoddy then (if I survive the fall) I can sue the supplier. In other words, I can take risks with myself, but others should be prevented from exposing me to undue levels of risk. Even if I wished to consent to purchasing a poor quality piece of equipment, that should not absolve the manufacturer or supplier from responsibility and regulations, safety standards and so on exist to protect the foolhardy from the designs of others.

If we transpose this argument to the research ethics context, the researcher is in an analogous position to the manufacturer of my climbing harness. If I expose myself to various procedures on my own behalf, it is my autonomous right to do so, but if I altruistically volunteer to expose myself to procedures set up by another as part of research, there should be regulations in place to limit the extent of the risk to which I may consent. As Savulescu reminds us, people will offer themselves for the most extraordinary situations: 'After all, one healthy person offered his own heart when Barney Clark received the first artificial heart!' (2001: 150). We can thus bring together the issues of consent and protection and say that, as long as there are proper safeguards to prevent student researchers designing projects that carry an expected risk of harm, and as long as there is a sound educational basis to the project, there should be no ethical bar to recruitment even if the probability of the discovery of new knowledge is slight.

Finally, to bring the argument back to respect and protection: we should respect the right of the would-be research participant to offer his or her services to the student researcher by ensuring fully informed consent, including the fact that the objective of the research is educational rather than the generation of new knowledge in the field. At the same time we should ensure that the participant is protected by ensuring that student projects do not offer any expected risk or chance of harm. Given that there may be some benefits to the participant in taking part, perhaps through the personal satisfaction of helping in professional education, we might further argue that unreasonably to prevent willing volunteers from offering their services would itself be unethical. There is an analogous situation here with patients in the health service. Those training to be health-care professionals have always learned their trades by being allowed to practise on real patients. Teaching hospitals routinely inform patients that students are trained in the institution and patients can ask not to be exposed to students if they wish. The great majority of patients, however, far from expressing reservations about being used in this way willingly submit themselves for example to repeated examinations by students because they obtain some satisfaction from being able to help, from giving something back to the institution that has cared for them.[9]

Further remarks on researchers' duty to provide benefit and the question of obligation to volunteer

There is an interesting further slant to this: arguing from the perspective of health-care research, Harris (2005) has argued that there is in certain circumstances a moral obligation on members of the public to take part in medical research. Would it be possible to extend this argument to participation in student projects? Harris develops his argument from two basic principles. First, he suggests that the principle 'do no harm' leads us to conclude that:

> Where our actions will, or may probably prevent serious harm then if we can reasonably (given the balance of risk and burden to ourselves and benefit to others) we clearly should act because to fail to do so is to accept responsibility for the harm that then occurs.
>
> (Harris, 2005: 242)

We have a basic moral obligation to help other people in need, so where research is a means of relieving need there is a moral obligation that we should support such research. Harris's second argument is one of fairness and the problem of the 'free rider'. In the context of health care, we all receive important benefits from medical research – as Harris points out many of us would not have survived infancy but for the reduction in maternal and infant mortality achieved by medicine – and any of us may require life-saving treatment at some point in the future. If we are happy to receive the benefit from such research it would seem unfair if we were, however, to refuse to do anything to support further research.

It is perhaps stretching the point too far to suggest that the same moral obligation to support cancer research would also place the same heavy moral responsibility on us to support student projects in exercise or sports sciences. However, precisely the same arguments can be made, albeit without the same sense of import or urgency. If we accept that the education of those who are to work in sports and exercise science serves a public good, and if training and practical experience in research is a useful part of that education, then to obstruct such research is to obstruct the creation of the public good. If we remember that there is increasing recognition of the value of exercise in, for example, the treatment of depression, hypertension and obesity, then we are talking not just about feeding the narcissistic impulses of the body builder but making a significant contribution to health care. Thus Harris's first point, of not doing harm, can certainly be applied. Given the incidence of hypertension and depression in society we can also say with some confidence that we or those close to us are almost certainly going to experience one of these conditions and may very well benefit from programmes of management that involve exercise rather than medication. Harris's second argument, from fairness, also comes into play.

Premises 4 and 5 of our would-be argument above (see pp. 184–5), simply state that participation in research involves certain risks or costs, but that these can be justified if they are proportionate to the expected benefit of the research. This seems uncontroversial but of course requires that we attempt to define and quantify the risks and benefits, and agree that they are proportionate. If the benefit of a student project is of the somewhat tentative nature that we have suggested, offering educational benefit and thus contributing to a public good in a rather tenuous way, then clearly any risks or costs must be minimal. As we have seen, this proportionality cuts deeper with academics whose research genuinely entails risks, even where risks are not expected but are possible, as was the case with early heart replacement research (Shephard, 2002).

The sixth premise states that scientifically invalid research offers no prospect of benefit. As we have already argued at some length, the scientific outcome of the project is not the only form of morally relevant benefit, so we can challenge the truth of the premise, simply saying that there are benefits to be obtained from the conduct of even small projects from which one cannot generate generalisable knowledge. Thus certain kinds of scientifically invalid research may yet offer benefit. The important distinction here concerns the intention behind the project. If researchers design a large-scale study purporting to offer great scientific benefit, obtain funding for it and recruit large numbers of participants, but their design is so flawed as to render the results meaningless, then clearly there will be little benefit. Also, the ethics of the project could be questioned – as noted above – in terms of wasting resources, such as direct funding, misuse of time and so on. One might argue that, if a lesson was learned and future trials are better designed, then there has been some benefit, but this will be minimal and probably will not justify the risks and costs associated with the project. This might well act as a corrective to the well-known publishers' bias towards positive reporting.

Ethical research and review: a tentative conclusion

So our argument – and our book – reaches its conclusion: does scientifically invalid research render it, *ipso facto*, unethical. We argue that this is not necessarily the case: the conclusion does not follow from the premises. We have shown that, in certain cases, the benefit from small-scale studies is educational rather than scientific, but that the education of professionals in research methods is in the public interest and serves the public good.

In order to provide a very loose standard to which researchers might be held accountable in the ethical and epistemological dimensions of their research we proposed the following:

1   Research involving human participants/subjects is ethically justifiable only if it holds out some realistic prospect of benefit.
2   Participation in research may involve risks or costs to the participants.
3   Such risks or costs are ethically justifiable so long as they are proportionate to the importance or benefit of the research.
4   Relevant benefits from research include the production of new knowledge and the education of future professionals and researchers, among other things.

5   Research projects that are unable to produce generalisable new know-
     ledge but that do offer other relevant benefits can be ethically justified,
     as long as the risks and costs are proportionate to that benefit.

We hope that in setting out some of the more significant abuses of research
we may also have alerted readers to some of the more mundane and everyday
errors and omissions. We hope too that our consideration of the key issues
of participation in research – as participant, researcher or subject – bring
with them ethical considerations that will come to be thought of as just one
more crucial ingredient of research design not merely the icing on the cake.

Notes

Introduction

1 On our account the word 'science' is not to be reserved only for experimental studies, as is the fashion among many laboratory-based scientists. We take our cue from the German concept *Wissenschaft*, which denotes any body of systematic and methodically derived knowledge. See McNamee (2005) for an elaboration of the philosophical thinking behind this conception and the undermining of 'the scientific method'.

1 Why does research need to be regulated? A selective history of research ethics abuses

1 See for example Homan (2002, 2005). The use of the term 'subject' or 'participant' is a hotly debated one. See Chapter 10 for a fuller discussion of this dispute.
2 These categories are taken from the Roith Report for the PCFC (PCFC, 1995) and have gained a measure of acceptance throughout higher education in the UK. A more up-to-date classification was published by the Parliamentary Office of Science and Technology (Postnote, 2005) which lists the following types of research involving humans: *biomedical* research, a general term for work in fields like medicine, genetics, physiology or biochemistry, that may involve research on people (e.g. gene therapy). A subdivision of this is *clinical research*, often concerned with the development of a drug, medical device or new surgical technique. *Clinical trials* are a specific type of clinical research in which new medicines or therapies undergo testing on humans to assess their efficacy, safety and quality. *Social science research* is concerned with the study of human society and relationships. *Psychological research*, mostly concerned with the study of individuals, may overlap clinical and social science research in its approach. It extends from the society-orientated spectrum of social psychology to the individual-orientated focus of experimental psychology. In addition, social care and health services research may need special scrutiny because they can involve vulnerable research subjects such as children or the mentally ill. This list is too sketchy but serves as a useful shorthand.
3 Note that the term 'clinical research' is taken by the World Medical Association to be synonymous with therapeutic, while 'non-clinical biomedical research' refers to non-therapeutic research.
4 See the extended discussion in Homan (2005) but also Bridges (2002) in the context of educational research. More generally, see the British Sociological Association's guidelines on the terminology of 'subject' and 'participant' (http://www.britsoc.co.uk/equality/63.htm).
5 See http://www.hhs.gov/ohrp/humansubjects/guidance/45cfr46.htm, accessed

7 March 2006: minimal risk means that: 'the probability and magnitude of harm or discomfort anticipated in the reasearch are not greater than those ordinarily encountered in daily life or during the performance of routine physical or psychological examinations or tests'.

6 Taken from Lord Russell of Liverpool (1954) *The Scourge of the Swastika* (Ballantine Books), cited in Godlovitch (1997).

7 For a fuller discussion of this case see Rothman and Rothman (1984).

8 However, it is worth noting that the Medical Research Council (MRC) in the UK now considers the distinction between therapeutic and non-therapeutic research to be unhelpful; see MRC 2004 Guidelines (www.mrc.ac.uk/pdf-ethics_ guide_ children.pdf, accessed 27 June 2006). Given the widespread use of this distinction we still observe it here.

2 What's in a name? Ethics, ethical theories and research ethics

1 For an introductory exposition of Kant's thinking see Benn (1998: 91–110), or for a more developed Kantian account (though not strictly following Kant's original) see Gert (1988).

2 We have deliberately eschewed discussion of non-human animals in research throughout the text. For a discussion of such see Singer (1993).

3 Precisely how reductionist the principles approach is is a matter of some debate. Gillon (2003) goes as far as saying that the four together are all-encompassing – and that their application is likely to become further utilised beyond healthcare spheres – and that the principle of respect is the most important of them. He invokes the Roman idea *primus inter pares* (first among equals) to denote this idea.

4 A caveat is necessary, even at this late stage. Some research simply presents us with dilemmas where there are no blame-free or guilt-free options. Simply coming to know certain information can put us in a moral dilemma. For one discussion of this idea – very close to the political notion of 'dirty hands', see McNamee (2002).

3 Research governance: the ethics review and approval processes

1 In this chapter, the terms Research Ethics Committees and Institutional Review Boards are used interchangeably. Ethics committees in the USA serve to resolve dilemmas regarding patient care (clinical settings), but similarly named committees elsewhere serve the same function as IRBs do in the USA (research settings). Here, the two terms both refer to the process of research approval. Despite its clumsiness, we will refer to both at all times IRBs/RECs, thus.

2 For a full litany of the participation of doctors in the abuse of human rights, see BMA (1992).

3 An MREC member of our acquaintance recently bemoaned their attendance at a recent – and regular – eight-hour meeting. Speaking from a position of familiarity with such meetings, it must be said that this requires a prodigious feat of concentration if all proposals are to be heard critically and fairly.

4 For example, where specialist knowledge may be desirable, such as particular medical knowledge relating to pregnancy, when pregnant women are utilised as research subjects or participants.

5 Consider the following example. A collaborative study in two countries is proposed, where one committee failed to approve the project because a member did not agree with the proposed statistical analysis. The committee at the site of the investigation, however, may have glossed over the issue of obtaining written first-person consent from illiterate subjects who subscribe to a notion of community rather than individual rights – a more subtle ethical difficulty. See Chapter 4 for a more detailed discussion of this latter difficulty.

6 From personal correspondence with the author. By 'open section member' is meant a member not specifically aligned to the dominant sciences of exercise and sports (i.e. biomechanics, physiology or psychology sections).

7 Take, for example, the practice of requiring researchers to submit essentially the same information in different formats for different committees. While desirable from a committee point of view, it increases the administrative burden on researchers.

8 We acknowledge that most IRBs in the USA have policies that expedite the review process where research is classified as having minimal risk. This is by no means a worldwide procedure, however.

9 In the USA this is relatively common practice, but this is not necessarily the case elsewhere.

4 Respectful research: why 'tick-box consent' is not good enough

1 See, for example the *locus classicus* of the modern analyses of freedom in 'Two Concepts of Liberty' (in Berlin, 1968: 118–72).

2 This list has been adapted from the list of considerations made by Beauchamp and Childress (2001: 65) in relation to medical treatment.

3 Though, for a historical perspective in relation to behavioural research, see Kimmel (1996: 38).

4 Granted, it could be argued that the 'subjects' of say a maximal physiological experiment into lactate thresholds are never inert but always *qua* human being responding to their environment. We say a little more about this on p. 87 – better ethics can mean better data.

5 We will not discuss here the competence of the researcher to carry out the research but only the competence of the researched to give their informed consent.

6 We have grossly simplified a complex area here – even in the absence of considering special or vulnerable populations. See White (1992: esp. 44–81). In relation to health research see Beauchamp and Childress (2001: 70–77).

7 For further discussion of how the issue of excessive inducements are estimated see Kimmell (1996: 222–4), Korn and Hogan (1992) and also Blanck *et al.* (1992) on the use of assistants attractive to the potential participant to bring about more effective recruitment.

8 Beauchamp and Childress (2001) enumerate three standards. The first is the physician's own professional standard, what is called the Doctor's Own Standard, which for our purposes is ignored.

9 It should be noted that their research was based on research conducted in US medical schools. Nevertheless they go on to cite ten other recent studies which indicate a disparity between the readability of the informed consent forms and the abilities of the subjects.

6 Scientific misconduct: authorship, plagiarism and fraud, and blowing the whistle on it

1 For a US perspective on what those pressures to publish look like and their tendency to drive plagiarism, as well as a cursory note on the upward trend of scientific productivity see Woolf (1985).

2 For amplification of the story see Waller (2002: 222–45)

3 For richer insights into this troubled history see Gratzer (2002: 142–5).

4 One might also make an observation about justice-as-merit in the opposite direction. It is sometimes said that there is an inverse relation between the number of references and the amount of independent thought in an article. Clearly, it is

critical to reference appropriately to show that one's work can be located within (or against) a certain tradition or method. This can easily slide into ornamental referencing, which is inauthentic. One of the chief examples of this is the referencing of a classic source which the authors have neither seen nor read but know will be expected to follow a certain point. Perhaps the chief example of this in research methods is the citing of Thomas Kuhn after his classic work on paradigms in the early 1960s. The reference is 'always' to the classic text *The Nature and Structure of Scientific Revolutions* (1962). The frequency with which authors either misconceive what Kuhn meant (and thereby manifest their failure to have read him and thus have referenced him unjustly), or indeed fail to note that his views were significantly altered in later texts (see Kuhn, 2000), indicates a lack of first-hand knowledge of Kuhn's work.

5 Among many credible media sources on the story see: http://www.guardian.co.uk/ korea/article/0,,1673788,00.html, accessed 2 Feb. 2006.
6 Part of this section is derived from McNamee (2001).
7 The term 'salience' is used here in a technical sense – one that is established in the mainstream ethics literature. It refers to the ethical significance of certain features of a situation (others might say 'morally relevant features') that are perceived by an agent. See, for example, its use in the deontological writing of Herman (1993: 73–93) and in the Aristotelian writings of Sherman (1989: 44–50).
8 Davis asserts that the standard theory is attributable to De George (1990: 200–14)
9 Sieber (1998: 16–17) discusses this point under the description of the prevailing ethnocentrism of organizational culture.
10 Boisjoly (1998: 71–2.) lists an American 'Government Accountability Project' which lists standard organizational responses:

   i) make the whistleblower, instead of the message, the issue;
   ii) isolate the whistleblower from the mainstream organization to a bureaucratic Siberia;
   iii) set the whistleblower up for a visible fall – the more obvious the better;
   iv) destabilize the whistleblower's support base;
   v) make outrageous charges against the whistleblower;
   vi) eliminate the whistleblower's job;
   vii) make the whistleblower struggle for self-preservation or career, family, finance and sanity.

11 It should be noted that if one does not blow the whistle, the possibility still exists for 'controlled leakage' (Eraut, 1984) where the researcher who is about to report publicly on an aspect of the research allows those who are its subject to have awareness of some portion or description of the research. One might further ask whether she could blow the whistle now or later, publicly or anonymously. These too should be considered in order to arrest the situation.
12 This entire volume of the *British Medical Journal* (1998, vol. 316) is worth reading on research misconduct from international perspectives.

7 Ethics in qualitative research

1 This chapter is not the appropriate place for a full debate on this particular ethical problem. Nevertheless, it would be remiss not to give an indication of what ought to be done and what ought to have been done at the review and proposal preparation stages. Very briefly, the imperative is to act. In this case, an appropriate authority must be notified. The notion of confidentiality is not absolute, and considerations of harm to the individual, possible harm to others and the potential inability of

the individual to act on her own behalf, all combine to override confidentiality in this instance. Clearly, referral to such agencies or authorities should have been signalled in the consent form/process and should have been noted at review stage by the appropriate IRB/REC.

2 For guidelines on the comprehensibility of informed consent forms, see Olivier and Olivier (2001).

3 This is not to suggest that covert methods are required necessarily for such research. Alternative, overt, methods may be possible without epistemic loss (see Gerrish, 1999).

4 Typing the words 'winner, Eddie, 1986, big wave' into a popular search engine resulted in a site that identifies Clyde Aikau, with the source site being http://holoholo.org/quikeddy/qhistory.html (accessed 7 May 2004).

5 Eddie refers to the Eddie Aikau Invitational, the premier big wave event held annually to celebrate the life of Clyde's late brother, who died in the ocean while trying to save his boat's crew.

8 Research ethics and vulnerable populations

1 Some material of this chapter is drawn from Edwards and McNamee (2005) *Journal of Medical Ethics* 31: 351–4, and is reproduced here with permission from the BMJ Publishing Group. We are grateful to Steve Edwards for his kind permission to use it and and also to the Soren Holm, editor of the *Journal of Medical Ethics*.

2 In Armstrong and van Mechelen's (2000) leading text on paediatric exercise physiology, there is not even a discussion of ethics.

3 Much of the section critical of these professional codes draws upon Edwards and McNamee (2005).

4 Nevill (2003) offers a useful practical guide here.

5 Equally, if we want to investigate the issue of child abuse in sport we may well have to explore the motivations of child abusers in sports, we must identify the paedophilial predators themselves (Brackenridge, 2001; Bringer; 2002) and this can only be done (since none are likely to volunteer their participation) with captive populations such as prisoners as well. Though in this particular instance a whole host of other related ethical issues rear their ugly heads.

6 Taking blood directly from the vein of a participant/subject.

7 We are grateful to Julien Baker, Bruce Davies and Ceri Nicholas respectively for the examples.

9 Does one size fit all? Ethics in transcultural research

1 We will explore community involvement in research design, initiation, approval, conduct and follow-up later in the chapter. We will also discuss the role of the community, as opposed to the individual, in decision-making.

2 With apologies to Shakespeare's Lady Macbeth and her physician.

3 We recognise that this is a gross generalisation, and that there are profound cultural differences not only with Africa, but within countries in Africa. Also, cultural boundaries are not rigidly defined and individuals can belong to multiple cultural groups. Nevertheless, the generalisation is a useful one, not only because it is reasonably accurate, but also because it serves to illustrate the points that we attempt to make.

4 It is probably worth noting that given the historical marginalisation of women in most societies, this is more likely to be a 'his' than a 'her'.

5 The construction of this narrative was inspired by the example of Ntombi, in Benatar (2002).

6 This of course discounts the view that any loss of liberty, caused by lack of

knowledge and the subsequent limitation on freedom of choice, constitutes a significant harm. It would be interesting to pursue precisely whether a utilitarian theory could make such a calculation in principle. For a critical view of such a view see Taylor (1985: 230–47) on incommensurable goods.

10 Research and society: is bad science *ipso facto* bad ethics?

1 The relationship between mainstream medicine – or at least medicine as tradition-ally conceived – and sports medicine is not a straightforward one. For a robust challenge to the sports medicine community see Edwards and McNamee (2006)
2 On this broader understanding of 'science' and related issues see McNamee (2005: 4–14).
3 After Boorse's classic essay 'Health as a Theoretical Concept' (1977).
4 The summary, though consistent with much of what has been discussed so far, is attributable to Benatar (2002).
5 For an extended discussion of research that was not, in hindsight, acceptable to the researched see Tickle (2002).
6 Though possibly not IRBs who often pass through without review 'standard edu-cational field tests' or research of a similar nature. We are aware that it is not wise to generalise too far here.
7 Of course the interpretation of that easily written phrase is not insignificant in itself!
8 See Illich (1973, 1975, 1977) for a trenchant critique of what he calls 'disabling professions' and Friedson (2001) for a more sympathetic account.
9 We do not deny the possibility that some participants might of course 'agree' because of perceived power differentials of the kind discussed by Kelman (1972). They might feel subtly coerced, or might fear some sort of sanction attached to non-participation. See Chapter 4 for a full discussion on conditions of informed consent, especially concerning power and voluntariness.

References

Ackerman T. F. (1989) 'An Ethical Framework for the Practice of Paying Research Subjects', *IRB* 11: 1–4.

ACHRE (Advisory Committee on Human Radiation Experiments) (n.d.) Final Report. URL: http://www.eh.doegov/ohre/roadmap/achre/index.html, accessed 28 Jan. 2006.

ACSM (American College of Sports Medicine) (2006) 'Exercise Testing for Children and Elderly People', in *Guidelines for Exercise Testing and Prescription*, 7th edn. London: Lippincott, Williams and Wilkins, pp. 237–51.

Alderson, P. (1992) 'Did Children Change or the Guidelines?', *Bulletin of Medical Ethics* 80: 21–8.

Allen-Collinson, J. (2005) 'Autoethnography: Self-Indulgence or Rigorous Methodology?', in M. McNamee (ed.) *Philosophy and the Sciences of Exercise, Health and Sport*. London: Routledge, pp. 187–202.

Al-Marzouki, S., Roberts, I., Marshall, T. and Evans, S. (2005) 'The Effect of Scientific Misconduct on the Results of Clinical Trials: A Delphi Survey', *Contemporary Clinical Trials* 26(3): 331–7.

Almond, B. (1993) 'Rights', in P. Singer (ed.) *A Companion to Ethics*. Oxford: Blackwell.

Alten, J. and Mariscalco, M. M. (2003) 'Critical Appraisal of Perez et al.: Jugular Venous Oxygen Saturation or Arteriovenous Difference of Lactate Content and Outcome in Children with Severe Traumatic Brain Injury', *Pediatric Critical Care Medicine* 4(1): 33–8.

Andersen, M. B. (2005) ' "Yeah, I Work with Beckham": Issues of Confidentiality, Privacy and Privilege in Sport Psychology Service and Delivery', *Sport and Exercise Psychology Review* 1(2): 3–13.

Annas, G. J. (1991) 'Ethics Committees: From Ethical Comfort to Ethical Cover', *The Hastings Center Report* 21: 18–21.

Annas, G. and Grodin, M. A. (eds) (1992) *The Nazi Doctors and the Nuremberg Code*. Oxford: Oxford University Press.

APA (American Psychological Association) (2002) *Ethical Principles of Psychologists and Code of Conduct*. URL: http://www.apa.org/ethics/cod2002.html#8_05, accessed 27 June 2006.

Aristotle (1998) *Nichomachaean Ethics*, trans W. D. Ross. Oxford: Oxford University Press.

Armstrong, N. and van Mechelen, W. (2000) *Paediatric Exercise Science and Medicine*. Oxford: Oxford University Press.

Arras, J. D. (2001) 'A Case Approach', in H. Kuhse and P. Singer (eds) *A Companion to Bioethics*. Oxford: Blackwell, pp. 106–15.

Ashcroft, R. (2003) 'The Ethics and Governance of Medical Research: What Does Regulation Have to Do with Morality?', *New Review of Bioethics* 1: 41–58.

Ashcroft, R. *et al.* (2005) 'Reforming Research Ethics Committees', *British Medical Journal* 331: 557–8.

Azar, B. (2002) 'Ethics at the Cost of Research?', *Monitor on Psychology* 33(2). URL: http://www.apa.org/monitor/feb02/ethicscost.html, accessed July 2006.

Baier, A. C. (1985) *Postures of the Mind*. London: Methuen.

Baier, A. C. (1993) *Moral Prejudices*. Boston, MA: Harvard University Press.

Banatvala, J. E. (1995) 'Unlinked Anonymous HIV Screening Programme in England and Wales', *British Medical Journal* 310: 206–7.

Barnes, D. M., Davis, A. J., Moran, T., Portillo, C. J. and Koenig, B. A. (1998) 'Informed Consent in a Multicultural Cancer Patient Population: Implications for Nursing Practice', *Nursing Ethics* 5(5): 412–23.

BASES (British Association of Sport and Exercise Sciences) (2000) *Code of Conduct*. URL: http://www.bases.org.uk/newsite/pdf/Code%20of%20Conduct.pdf, accessed 16 Feb. 2005.

Batty, D. (2003) 'Q&A: Data Protection and the Police', *The Guardian*, 18 Dec. URL: http://www.guardian.co.uk/soham/story/0,,1109845,00.html, accessed 16 Feb. 2006.

Bayles, M. D. (1988) 'The Professional–Client Relationship', in J. C. Callahan (ed.) *Ethical Issues in Professional Life*. Oxford: Oxford University Press, pp. 113–23.

BBC News (2004) 'Naked Rambler Completes his Trek', URL: http://news.bbc.co.uk/1/hi/scotland/3420685.stm, accessed 28 Jan. 2006.

Beauchamp, T. L. and Childress J. F. (1979) *Principles of Biomedical Ethics*, 1st edn. Oxford: Oxford University Press.

Beauchamp, T. L., Childress J. F. (2001) *Principles of Biomedical Ethics*, 5th edn. Oxford: Oxford University Press.

Bellah, R., Madsen, R., Sullivan, W., Swidler, A. and Tipton, S. (1985) *Habits of the Heart: Individualism and Commitment in American Life*. Berkeley, CA: University of California Press.

Belmont Report (1979) *Ethical Principles and Guidelines for the Protection of Human Subjects of Research*. DHEW (Department of Health, Education, and Welfare): National Commission for the Protection of Human Subjects of Biomedical and Behavioral Research.

Benatar, S. R. (2002) 'Reflections and Recommendations on Research Ethics in Developing Countries', *Social Science and Medicine* 54: 1131–41.

Bencko, V. (1996) 'Informed Consent in the Czech Republic', *The Science of the Total Environment* 184: 77–81.

Benn, P. (1998) *Ethics*. London: UCL Press.

Bensman, J. (1988) 'The aesthetics and politics of footnoting', *Politics, Culture and Society* 1: 443–70.

Bentham, J. (1948) *An Introduction to the Principles of Morals and Legislation*. New York: Macmillan.

Bentham, J. (1995) *The Panopticon Writings*, edited by M. Bozovic. London: Verso.

Bentley, J. P. and Thacker, P. G. (2004) 'The Influence of Risk and Monetary Payment on the Research Participation Decision Making Process', *Journal of Medical Ethics* 30: 293–8.

Berlin, I. (1968) *Four Essays on Liberty*. Oxford: Oxford University Press.

Beyrer, C. and Kass, N. E. (2002) 'Human Rights, Politics and Reviews of Research Ethics', *The Lancet* 360(9349).

Biddle, S. J., Bull, S. J. and Seheult, C. L. (1992) 'Ethical and Professional Issues in Contemporary British Sports Psychology', *The Sports Psychologist* 6: 66–76.

Biddle, S., Markland, Gilbourne, Chatzisrantis and Sparkes (2001) 'Research Methods in Sport and Exercise Science: Quantitative and Qualitative Issues', *Journal of Sports Sciences* 19: 777–809.

Blanck, P. D. *et al.* (1992) 'Scientific Rewards and Conflicts of Ethical Choices in Human Subjects Research', *American Psychologist* 47: 959–65.

Blum, L. (1993) *Moral Perception and Particularity*. Cambridge: Cambridge University Press.

BMA (British Medical Association) (1992) *Medicine Betrayed*. London: Zed Books.

Bogen, J. (2001) 'Experiment and Observation', in P. Machamer and M. Silberstein (eds) *The Blackwell Companion to the Philosophy of Science*. Oxford: Blackwell, pp. 128–48.

Bok, S. (1978a) 'Freedom and Risk', *Proceedings of the American Academy of Arts and Sciences* 107: 115–27.

Bok, S. (1978b) *Lying: Moral Choice in Public and Private Life*. New York: Quartet.

Bok, S. (1988) 'Whistleblowing and Professional Responsibilities', in J. Callahan (ed.) *Ethical Issues and Professional Life*. Oxford: Oxford University Press, pp. 331–9.

Boorse, C. (1977) 'Health as a Theoretical Concept', *Philosophy of Science* 44: 542–73.

Borchert, D. M. and Stewart, D. (1986) *Exploring Ethics*. New York: Macmillan.

Boisjoly, R. (1998), in J. E. Callahan (ed.) *Ethical Issues in Professional Life*. Oxford: Oxford University Press.

Bower, R. and de Gasparis, P. (1978) *Ethics in Social Research: Protecting the Interests of Human Subjects*. New York: Praeger.

BPA (British Paediatric Association) (1992) *Guidelines for the Ethical Conduct of Medical Research Involving Children*. London: BPA.

Brackenridge, C. (2001) *Spoilsports: Understanding and Preventing Sexual Exploitation in Sport*. London: Routledge.

Brazier, M. and Lobjoit, M. (eds) (1991) *Protecting the Vulnerable*. London: Routledge.

Brewer, J. D. (2000) *Ethnography*. Milton Keynes: Open University Press.

Bridges, D. (2001) 'The Ethics of Outsider Research', *Journal of the Philosophy of Education* 35(3): 371–86. Reprinted in M. McNamee and D. Bridges (eds) *The Ethics of Educational Research*. Oxford: Blackwell, 2002, pp. 71–88.

Bringer, J. D. (2002) 'Sexual Exploitation: Swimming Coaches' Perceptions and the Development of Role Conflict and Role Ambiguity', unpublished doctoral thesis, University of Gloucestershire.

Bringer, J. D., Brackenridge, C. H. and Johnston, L. H. (2002) 'Defining Appropriateness in Coach–Athlete Relationships: The Voice of Coaches', *Journal of Sexual Aggression* 8(2): 83–98.

Brodie, D. A. and Stopani, K. (1990) 'Experimental Ethics in Sports Medicine Research', *Sports Medicine* 9(3): 143–50.

Capron, A. M. (1989) 'Human Experimentation', in R. M. Veatch (ed.) *Medical Ethics*. Boston, MA: Jones and Bartlett Publishers, pp. 125–72.

Cardinal, B. J. (2000) '(Un)Informed Consent in Exercise and Sport Science Research? A Comparison of Forms Written for Two Reading Levels', *Research Quarterly for Exercise and Sport* 71: 295–301.

Cardinal, B. J., Martin, J. J. and Sachs, M. L. (1996) 'Readability of Written Informed

Consent Forms Used in Exercise and Sport Psychology Research', *Research Quarterly for Exercise and Sport* 67(3): 360–2.

Cardon, P. V., Dommel, F. W., Trumble, P. R. (1976) 'Injuries to Research Subjects: A Survey of Investigators', *New England Journal of Medicine* 295: 650–4.

Carrington, B., Chivers, T. and Williams, T. (1987) 'Gender, Leisure and Sport: A Case-Study of Young People of South Asian Descent', *Leisure Studies* 6: 265–79.

Casarett, D.J., Karlawish, J.H.T. and Moreno, J.D. (2002) 'A Taxonomy of Value in Clinical Research', *IRB* 24(6): 1–6.

Cashmore, E. (1982) 'Black Youth for Whites', in E. Cashmore and B. Troyna (eds.) *Black Youth in Crisis*. London: George Allen and Unwin, pp. 10–14.

Cashmore, E. and Troyna, B. (1981) 'Just for White Boys? Elitism, Racism and Research', *Multiracial Education* 10(1): 43–8.

Charlton, J. I. (1998) *Nothing About Us Without Us: Disability, Oppression and Empowerment*. London: University of California Press.

Christakis, N. A. (1992) 'Ethics Are Local: Engaging Cross-Cultural Variation in the Ethics for Clinical Research', *Social Science and Medicine* 35(9): 1079–91.

CIOMS (Council for International Organizations of Medical Sciences) (2002) *International Ethical Guidelines for Biomedical Research Involving Human Subjects*. URL: http://www.cioms.ch/frame_guidelines_nov_2002.htm, accessed July 2006.

Clarke, G. (1997) 'Playing a Part: The Lives of Lesbian Physical Education Teachers', in B. Humberstone (ed.) *Researching Women and Sport*. London: Macmillan, pp. 36–49.

Crigger, N. J., Holcomb, L. and Weiss, J. (2001) 'Fundamentalism, Multiculturalism and Problems of Conducting Research with Populations in Developing Nations', *Nursing Ethics* 8(5): 459–68.

Crosby, S. and Grodin, M. A. (2002) 'The Challenges of Cross-Cultural Research in the International Setting', *Ethics and Behaviour Forum* 12(4): 376–8.

Crossett, T. (1995) *Outsiders in the Clubhouse: The World of Women's Professional Golf*. Albany, NY: SUNY Press.

Culver, C. M. and Gert, B. (1982) *Philosophy and Medicine*. Oxford: Oxford University Press.

D'Agostino, F. (1995) 'The Ethics of Social Research', *Journal of Applied Philosophy* 12(1): 65–76.

Davis, M. (1996) 'Some Paradoxes of Whistleblowing', *Business and Professional Ethics Journal* 15(1): 3–21.

Dawson, A. J. (2004) 'Methodological Reasons for not Gaining Prior Informed Consent Are Sometimes Justified', *British Medical Journal* 329: 87.

Dawson, N. and L. Kass L (2005) 'Views of US Researchers about Informed Consent in International Collaborative Research', *Social Science and Medicine* 61(6): 1211–22.

De George, R. T. (1990) *Business Ethics*, 3rd edn. New York: Macmillan.

Department of Health (2001) *Governance Arrangements for Research Ethics Committees*. London: Department of Health.

DHHS (Department of Heath and Human Services) (2005) *Code of Federal Regulations: Protection of Human Subjects*. URL: http://www.hhs.gov/ohrp/humansubjects/guidance/45cfr46.htm, accessed 7 March 2006.

Dickert, N. and Grady, C. (1999) 'What's the Price of a Research Subject? Approaches to Payment for Research Participation', *New England Journal of Medicine* 341: 198–203.

Diener, E. and Crandall, R. (1978) *Ethics in Social and Behavioral Research*. Chicago, IL: University of Chicago Press.

Drowatzky, J. N. (1996) *Ethical Decision Making in Physical Activity Research*. Champaign, IL: Human Kinetics.

Dworkin, G. (1983) 'Paternalism', in R. Sartorius (ed) *Paternalism*. Minneapolis, MN: University of Minnesota Press, pp. 19–34.

Dyer, C. (1997) 'Consultant Struck Off Over Research Fraud', *British Medical Journal* 315: 205–10.

Dyer, O. (2003) 'GMC Reprimands Doctor for Research Fraud', *British Medical Journal* 326: 730.

Eaton, L. (2004) 'A Quarter of UK Students are Guilty of Plagiarism, Survey Shows', *British Medical Journal* 329: 70.

Edwards, S. D. (2000) 'An Argument against Research on People with Intellectual Disabilities', *Medicine, Health Care and Philosophy* 3: 69–73.

Edwards, S. D. and McNamee, M. J. (2005) 'Ethical Concerns Regarding Guidelines for the Conduct of Clinical Research on Children', *Journal of Medical Ethics* 31: 351–4.

Edwards, S. D. and McNamee, M. J. (2006) 'Sports Medicine Is Not Medicine', *Health Care Analysis*.

Edwards, S. J. L., Kirchin, S. and Huxtable, R. (2004) 'Research Ethics Committees and Paternalism', *Journal of Medical Ethics* 30: 88–91.

Elias, N. (1978) *The Civilizing Process: The History of Manners*. New York: Urizen.

Embassy of France in the US (2005) 'French Legislation on Privacy'. URL: http://www.ambafrance-us.org/atoz/privacy.asp, accessed 28 Jan. 2006.

Eraut, M. (1984) 'Institution-Based Curriculum Evaluation', in M. Skilbeck (ed.) *Evaluating the Curriculum in the Eighties*. London: Hodder and Stoughton.

ESRC (Economic and Social Research Council) (2006) *Research Ethics Framework*. URL: http://www.esrc.ac.uk/ESRCInfoCentre/Images/ESRC_Re_Ethics_Frame_tcm6-11291.pdf, accessed 28 Jan. 2006.

Evans, D. and Evans, M. (1996) *A Decent Proposal: Ethical Review of Clinical Research*. Chichester: Wiley.

Faden, R. R., King, N. M. P. and Beauchamp, T. L. (1986) *History of Informed Consent*. Oxford: Oxford University Press.

Fairchild, A. and Bayer, R. (1999) 'The Uses and Abuses of Tuskegee', *Science* 284(5416): 919–21.

Feinberg, J. (1983) 'Legal Paternalism', in R. Sartorius (ed.) *Paternalism*. Minneapolis, MN: University of Minnesota Press, pp. 3–18.

Fethe, C. (1993) 'Beyond Voluntary Consent: Hans Jonas on the Moral Requirements of Human Experimentation', *Journal of Medical Ethics* 19: 99–103.

Fine, G. (1987) *With the Boys: Little League Baseball and Preadolescent Culture*. Chicago, IL: University of Chicago Press.

Fishwick, L. (1983) 'Cohesion in Interacting Sports: A Preliminary Qualitative Study Using Three Women's Teams', unpublished MSc thesis, Dalhousie University.

Fishwick, L. (1990) 'A Sporting Chance? Resegregation of Coaching Jobs in Women's Intercollegiate Athletics', unpublished PhD thesis, University of Illinois.

Flynn, S., Dixon, C., Amos, T. and Appleby, L. (2000) 'The Cost of Getting Approval', *British Medical Journal* 320(7243): 1183.

Foucault, M. (1995) *Discipline and Punish: The Birth of the Prison*. New York: Vintage Books.

French, E. (1987) 'The Political Aspect of Research Ethics in the Human Sciences', *South African Journal of Sociology* 18(1): 14–21.

Friedson, E. (2001) *Professionalism: The Third Logic*. Cambridge: Polity.

Gadlin, H. (1998) 'Can You Whistle While You Work?', *Science and Engineering Ethics* 4: 65–9.

Gerrish, K. (1999) 'Inequalities in Service Provision', *Journal of Advanced Nursing* 30(6): 1263–71.

Gert, B. (1988) *Morality*. Oxford: Oxford University Press.

Gibson, W. (2003) *Pattern Recognition*. London: Penguin.

Gilligan, C. (1982) *In a Different Voice*. Boston, MA: Harvard University Press.

Gillon, R. (1991) 'Research on the Vulnerable: An Ethical Overview', in M. Brazier and M. Lobjoit (eds) *Protecting the Vulnerable*. London: Routledge, pp. 52–76.

Gillon, R. (2003) 'Ethics needs principles – four can encompass the rest – and respect for autonomy should be "first among equals" ', *Journal of Medical Ethics* 29: 307–12.

Girard, M. (1988) 'Technical Expertise as an Ethical Form: Towards an Ethics of Distance', *Journal of Medical Ethics* 14: 25–30.

Giulianotti, R. (1995) 'Participant Observation and Research into Football Hooliganism: Reflections on the Problems of Entree and Everyday Risks', *Sociology of Sport Journal* 12: 1–20.

Godlovitch, S. (1997) 'Forbidding Nasty Knowledge: On the Use of Ill Gotten Information', *Journal of Applied Philosophy* 14(1): 1–17.

Gomm, R. (2004) *Social Research Methodology*. London: Palgrave.

Gratzer, W. (2002) *Eurekas and Euphorbias*. Oxford: Oxford University Press.

Grinnel, F. (1997) 'Truth, Fairness and the Definition of Scientific Misconduct', *Journal of Laboratory and Clinical Medicine* 129.

Guest, S. (1997) 'Compensation for Subjects of Medical Research: The Moral Rights of Patients and the Power of Research Ethics Committees', *Journal of Medical Ethics* 23: 181–5.

Guidelines for Exercise Testing and Prescription (ACSM) (2006). London: Lippincott, Williams and Wilkins.

Hannigan, B. and Allen, D. (2003) 'A Tale of Two Studies: Research Governance Issues Arising from Two Ethnographic Investigations into the Organisation of Health and Social Care', *International Journal of Nursing Studies* 40: 685–95.

Harris, J. (2005) 'Scientific Research is a Moral Duty', *Journal of Medical Ethics* 31: 242–8.

Harth, S. C. and Thong, Y. H. (1995) 'Aftercare for participants in clinical research: ethical considerations in an asthma drug trial', *Journal of Medical Ethics* 21(4): 225–8.

Hebestreit, H. U. and Bar-Or, O. (2005) 'Differences between Children and Adults for Exercise Testing and Exercise Prescription', in J. Skinner (ed.) *Exercise Testing and Exercise Prescription for Special Cases*, 3rd edn. London: Lippincott, Williams and Wilkins, pp. 68–84.

Herman, B. (1993) *The Practice of Moral Judgement*. London: Harvard University Press.

Heyman, S. R. and Andersen, M. B. (1998) 'When to Refer Athletes for Counselling or Psychotherapy', in J. M. Williams (ed.) *Applied Sport Psychology*, 3rd edn. Mountain View, CA: Mayfield, pp. 359–71.

Hillman, H. (1998) 'Some Aspects Do not Fall in Remit of Bodies Examining Fraud', *British Medical Journal* 317: 1590.

Hipshman, L. (1999) 'Attitudes Towards Informed Consent, Confidentiality, and Substitute Treatment Decisions in Southern African Medical Students: A Case Study from Zimbabwe', *Social Science and Medicine* 49: 313–28.

Hoffman, D., Tarzian, A. and O'Neill, A. (2000) 'Are Ethics Committee Members Competent to Consult?', *Journal of Law, Medicine and Ethics* 28(1): 30.

Hoffmaster, B. (1992) 'Can Ethnography Save the Life of Medical Ethics?', *Social Science and Medicine* 35(12): 1421–31.

Homan, R. (1991) *The Ethics of Social Research*. London: Macmillan.

Homan, R. (2002) 'The Principle of Assumed Consent', in M. J. McNamee and D. Bridges (eds) *The Ethics of Educational Research*. Oxford: Blackwell, pp. 23–40.

Homan, R. (2005) 'Is Research on and with Students Ethically Defensible?', in M. J. McNamee (ed.) *Philosophy and the Sciences of Exercise, Health And Sport*. London: Routledge.

Hooey, J. (2000) 'Who Wrote this Paper Anyway? The New Vancouver Group Statement Refines the Definition of Authorship', *Canadian Medical Association Journal* 163(6): 1426–7.

Hume, D. (1978) *An Enquiry Concerning Human Nature*, edited by L. A. Selby-Bigge and P. A. Nidditch. Oxford: Clarendon Press.

Humphreys, L. (1970). *Tea Room Trade: Impersonal Sex in Public Places*. Chicago, IL: Aldine.

Ijsellmuiden, C. B. and Faden, R. R. (1992) 'Research and Informed Consent in Africa – Another Look', *New England Journal of Medicine* 326(12): 830–4.

Illich, I. (1973) *Deschooling Society*. Harmondsworth: Penguin.

Illich, I. (1975) *Medical Nemesis: The Expropriation of Health*. London: Marian Boyars.

Illich, I. (1977) *Disabling Professions*. London: Marion Boyars.

International Committee of Medical Journal Editors (2005) Uniform Requirements for Manuscripts Submitted to Biomedical Journals. URL: http://www.imje.org/imje.pdf, accessed 23 Jan. 2005.

Iversen, A., Liddell, K., Fear, N., Hotopf, M. and Wessely, S. (2006) 'Consent, Confidentiality and the Data Protection Act', *British Medical Journal* 332: 165–9.

Jacklin, P. B., Roberts J. A., Wallace P., Haines, A., Harrison, R., Barber, J. A. *et al.* (2003) 'Virtual Outreach: Economic Evaluation of Joint Teleconsultations for Patients Referred by their General Practitioner for a Specialist Opinion', *British Medical Journal* 327(7406): 84.

Jago, R. and Bailey, R. (2001) 'Ethics and Paediatric Exercise Science: Issues and Making a Submission to a Local Ethics and Research Committee', *Journal of Sports Sciences* 19: 527–35.

James, G. G. (1988) 'In Defense of Whistleblowing', in J. Callahan (ed.) *Ethical Issues in Professional Life*. Oxford: Oxford University Press, pp. 315–22.

Jones, C. R. (2005) 'Developing Good Practitioners: Issues of Clarification and Character', *Sport and Exercise Psychology Review* 2(2).

Jonsen, A. R. and Toulmin, S. E. (1988) *The Abuse of Casuistry: A History of Moral Reasoning*. Berkeley, CA: University of California Press.

Kabat, T. (1975) 'Ethics and the Wrong Answer', *Science* 189(4202): 505.

Kant, I. (1948 [1785]) 'Groundwork of the Metaphysic of Morals', in *The Moral Law*, ed. and trans. by H. J. Paton. London: Hutchinson.

Katz, J. (1993) ' "Ethics and Clinical Research" Revisited: A Tribute to Henry K. Beecher', *The Hastings Center Report* 23: 31–9.

Kelman, H. C. (1972) 'The Rights of the Subject in Social Research: An Analysis in Terms of Relative Power and Legitimacy', *American Psychologist* 27: 989–1016.

Kimmell, A. J. (1996) *Ethical Issues in Behavioural Research*. Oxford: Blackwell.

Kitsburg, A. (2001) 'Cribbage', *British Medical Journal* 322(27 Jan.): 226.

Klein, A. (1993) *Little Big Men: Bodybuilding Subculture and Gender Construction*. Albany, NY: SUNY Press.

Kleinig, J. (1984) *Paternalism*. Manchester: Manchester University Press.

Koestler, A. (1974) *The Case of the Midwife Toad*. London: Random House.

Kopelman, L. (2000) 'Children as Research Subjects: A Dilemma', *Journal of Medicine and Philosophy* 25(6): 745–64.

Korn, J. H. and Hogan, K. A. (1992) 'Effects of Incentives and Aversiveness of Treatment on Willingness to Participate in Research', *Teaching of Psychology* 19: 21–24.

Kottow, M. H. (2004) 'Vulnerability: What Kind of Principle Is It?', *Medicine, Health Care and Philosophy* 7: 281–7.

Kroll, W. (1993) 'Ethical Issues in Human Research', *Quest* 45(1): 32–44.

Kuczewski, M. and McCruden, P. J. (2001) 'Informed Consent: Does it Take a Village? The Problem of Culture and Truth Telling', *Cambridge Quarterly of Healthcare Ethics* 10: 34–46.

Kuhn, T. S. (1962) *The Nature and Structure of Scientific Revolutions*. Chicago, IL: University of Chicago Press.

Kuhn, T. S. (2000) *The Road Since Structure*. Chicago, IL: University of Chicago Press.

Kultgen, J. (1991) *Ethics and Professionalism*. Philadelphia, PA: University of Pennsylvania Press.

Kultgen, J. (1995) *Autonomy and Intervention: Parentalism in the Caring Life*. New York: Oxford University Press.

Lafollette, H. (ed.) (2000) *Blackwell Guide to Ethical Theory*. Oxford: Blackwell.

Lafollette, H. (ed.) (2002) *Ethics in Practice*. Oxford: Blackwell.

Lancet (1991) 'Informed Consent: How Informed?' (Editorial), *Lancet* 338(8768): 665–6.

Lancet (2001) 'Improving the Safety of Patients during Clinical Research' (Editorial), *Lancet* 357(9274): 2067.

Lawrence, E. (1981) 'White Sociology, Black Struggle', *Multiracial Education* 10(1): 3–17.

Leach, A., Hilton, S., Greenwood, B. M., Manneh, E., Dibba, B., Wilkins, A. and Mulholland, E. K. (1999) 'An Evaluation of the Informed Consent Procedure Used During a Trial of a *Haemophilus influenzae* Type B Conjugate Vaccine Undertaken in The Gambia, West Africa', *Social Science and Medicine* 48: 139–48.

Lehrer, T. (1953) 'Lobachevsky', released on *Songs by Tom Lehrer*. Lehrer Records.

Levine, C. *et al.* (2004) 'The limitations of "vulnerability" as a protection for human research participants', *American Journal of Bioethics* 4(3): 44.

Liemohn, W. (1979) 'Research Involving Human Subjects', *The Research Quarterly* 50(2): 157–64.

Lux, A. L., Edwards, S. W. and Osborne, J. P. (2000) 'Responses of Local Research Ethics Committees to a Study with Approval from a Multicentre Research Ethics Committee', *British Medical Journal* 320(7243): 1182.

Macilwain, C. (1996) 'Public Faith in Science Stays High', *Nature* 381: 355.

MacIntyre, A. C. (1984) *After Virtue: A Study in Moral Virtue*. London: Duckworth.

MacIntyre, A. C. (1986) *After Virtue: A Study in Moral Virtue*, 2nd edn. London: Duckworth.

MacIntyre, A. C. (1999) *Dependent Rational Animals: Why Human Beings Need the Virtues*. London: Duckworth.

Macklin, R. (1981) ' "Due" and "Undue" Inducements: On Paying Money to Research Subjects', *IRB* 3: 1–6.

Macklin R. (2003) 'Bioethics, Vulnerability, and Protection', *Bioethics* 17(5–6): 472–86.

McNamee, M. J. (1998) 'Celebrating Trust: Rules and Virtues in the Conduct of Coaches', in M. J. McNamee and S. J. Parry (eds) *Ethics and Sport*. London: Routledge, pp. 148–68.

McNamee, M. J. (2001) 'The Guilt of Whistling While You Work: Conflicts in Action Research and Educational Ethnography', *Journal of Philosophy of Education* 35(4): 423–41. Reprinted in M. J. McNamee and D. Bridges (eds) *The Ethics of Educational Research*. Oxford: Blackwell, 2002, pp. 128–50.

McNamee, M. J. (2005) 'Positivism, Popper and Paradigms', in M. J. McNamee (ed.) *Philosophy and the Sciences of Exercise, Health and Sport*. London: Routledge, pp. 1–25.

Mahon, J. (1987) 'Ethics in Drug Testing in Human Beings', in J. D. G. Evans (ed.) *Moral Philosophy and Contemporary Problems*. Cambridge: Cambridge University Press, pp. 199–211.

Marcus, J. (2004) 'Harvard Quizzed on Research Ethics', *Times Higher Educational Supplement* 28 May: 14.

Martin, B. (1994) 'Plagiarism: A Misplaced Emphasis', *Journal of Information Ethics* 3(2): 36–47.

Martinez, L. R. and Haymes, E. M. (1992) 'Substrate Utilization during Treadmill Running in Prepubertal Girls and Women', *Medicine and Science in Sports and Exercise* 24(9): 975–83.

Mill, J. S. (1962 [1863]) 'Utilitarianism', in M. Warnock (ed.) *Utilitarianism*. London: Fontana Press, pp. 251–321.

Mills, J. *et al.* (2005) 'Designing Research in Vulnerable Populations: Lessons from HIV Prevention Trials that Stopped Early', *British Medical Journal* 331: 1403–6.

Mitford, J. (1988) 'Cheaper than Chimpanzees', in J. Callahan (ed.) *Ethical Issues in Professional Life*. Oxford: Oxford University Press, pp. 189–93.

Morgan, R. E. (1974) *Concerns and Values in Physical Education*. London: Bell.

Morgan, D. L. and Kreuger, R. A. (1993) 'When to Use Focus Groups and Why', in D. L. Morgan (ed.) *Successful Focus Groups: Advancing the State of the Art*. London: Sage.

Mosher, D. L. (1988) 'Balancing the Rights of Subjects, Scientists, and Society: 10 Principles for Human Subject Committees', *The Journal of Sex Research* 24: 378–85.

MRC (Medical Research Council) (2000) *Personal Information in Medical Research* London: MRC.

MRC (Medical Research Council) (2004) *MRC Ethics Guide: Medical Research Involving Children*. URL: www.mrc.ac.uk/pdf-ethics_guide_children.pdf, accessed 27 June 2006.

Nagel, T. (1989) *The View from Nowhere*. Oxford: Oxford University Press.

NBAC (National Bioethics Advisory Committee) (1999) *Ethical Perspectives on the Research Use of Human Biological Materials*. Washington, DC: NBAC.

Nevill, M. (2003) 'Young People as Participants in Exercise Physiology Research: Practical Issues', *Journal of Sport Sciences* 28(1): 881.

Nicholson, R. G. (1986) *Medical Research with Children: Ethics, Law and Practice.* Oxford: Oxford University Press.

Oderberg, D. S. (2000) *Applied Ethics, A Non-Consequentialist Approach.* Oxford: Blackwell.

Ogilvie, R. I. (2001) 'The Death of a Volunteer Research Subject: Lessons to be Learned', *Canadian Medical Association Journal* 165: 1335–7.

Olivier, S. C. (1995) 'Ethical Considerations in Human Movement Research', *Quest* 47: 135–43.

Olivier, S. C. (1996) 'Rights, Obligations, and Utility in Sports Medicine Research', *South African Journal of Sports Medicine* 3(3): 19–22.

Olivier, S. C. (2002) 'Ethics Review of Research Projects Involving Human Subjects', *Quest* 54: 194–204.

Olivier, S. C. and Olivier, A. (2001) 'Comprehension in the Informed Consent Process', *Sportscience* 5(3). URL: www.sportsci.org.

O'Neill, O. (2002) *Autonomy and Trust in Bioethics.* Cambridge: Cambridge University Press.

O'Neill, O. (2003) 'Some Limits of Informed Consent', *Journal of Medical Ethics* 29: 4–7.

Orwell, G. (2000) *Nineteen Eighty-Four.* London: Penguin.

Paasche-Orlow, M. K. *et al.* (2003) 'Readability Standards for Informed-consent Forms as Compared with Actual Readability', *New England Journal of Medicine* 348: 721–6.

Parent, W. A. (1983) 'Privacy, Morality and the Law', *Philosophy and Public Affairs* 12(4): 269–88.

Parry, S. J. (2005) 'Must Scientists Think Philosophically about Science?', in M. J. McNamee (ed.) *Philosophy and the Sciences of Exercise, Health and Sport.* London: Routledge.

Patrick, J. M. (1983) 'Volunteers or Pressed Men: Human Subjects in Science', *Ergonomics* 26(7): 637–8.

Payne, S., Large, S., Jarrett, N. and Turner, P. (2000) 'Written Information Given to Patients and Families by Palliative Care Units: A National Survey', *The Lancet* 355(9217): 1792.

PCFC (Polytechnics and Colleges Funding Council) (1995) Roith Report. URL: http://www.hefce.ac.uk/pubs/hefce/1995/c10_95.htm, accessed 29 June 2006.

Peled, E. and Leichentritt, R. (2002) 'The Ethics of Qualitative Social Work Research', *Qualitative Social Work* 1(2): 145–69.

Pettit, P. (1992) 'Instituting a Research Ethic: Chilling and Cautionary Tales', *Bioethics* 6(2): 89–112.

Pincoffs, E. L. (1986) *Quandaries and Virtues.* Lawrence, KS: University of Kansas Press.

Postnote (2005) (Parliamentary Office for Science and Technology) no. 243, July.

Pownall, M. (1999) 'Falsifying Data is Main Problem in US Research Fraud Review', *British Medical Journal* 318: 1164.

Price, D. K. (1978) 'Endless Frontier or Bureaucratic Morass?', in G. Holton and R. S. Morrison (eds) *Limits of Scientific Inquiry.* New York: W. W. Norton, pp. 75–92.

Pronger, B. (1990) 'Gay Jocks: A Phenomenology of Gay Men in Athletics', in M. Messner and D. Sabo (eds) *Sport Men and the Gender Order.* Champaign, IL: Human Kinetics, pp. 141–52.

Punch, M. (1998) 'Politics and Ethics in Qualitative Research', in N. Denzin and Y. Lincoln (eds) *The Landscape of Qualitative Research: Theories and Issues*. London: Sage, pp. 156–84.

Rachels, J. (2001) 'Ethical Theory and Bioethics', in H. Kuhse, and P. Singer (eds) *A Companion to Bioethics*. Oxford: Blackwell.

Ramcharan, P. and Cutcliffe, J. (2001) 'Judging the Ethics of Qualitative Research: Considering the "Ethics as Process" Model', *Health and Social Care in the Community* 9(6): 358–66.

Ramsbottom, R. *et al.* (1994) 'Accumulated Oxygen Deficit and Short-Distance Running Performance', *Journal of Sports Sciences* 12: 447–53.

Ramsbottom, R. *et al.* (1997) 'Accumulated Oxygen Deficit and Shuttle Run Performance in Physically Active Men and Women', *Journal of Sports Sciences* 15: 207–14.

Rapport, F. (ed.) (2004) *New Qualitative Methodologies in Health and Social Care Research*. London: Routledge.

Rapport, F., Wainwright, P. and Elwyn, G. (2005) ' "Of the Edgelands": Broadening the Scope of Qualitative Methodology', *Medical Humanities* 31(1): 37–43.

Rashad, A. M., Phipps, F. M. and Haith-Cooper, M. (2004) 'Obtaining Informed Consent in an Egyptian Research Study', *Nursing Ethics* 11(4): 394–9.

Raval, S. (1989) 'Gender, Leisure and Sport: A Case Study of Young People of South Asian Descent – A Response', *Leisure Studies* 8: 237–40.

RCPCH (Royal College of Paediatrics and Child Health) (2000) 'Guidelines for the Ethical Conduct of Medical Research Involving Children', *Archives of Disease in Childhood* 82: 177–82.

Rennie, D. (1998) 'An American Perspective on Research Integrity', *British Medical Journal* 316 (7146): 1726–35.

Rex, J. (1981) 'Errol Lawrence and the Sociology of Race Relations: An Open Letter', *Multiracial Education* 10(1): 49–51.

Rifkin, J. (1988) 'Ethics in Embryo: A Symposium', *Dialogue* 3: 57–63.

Robling, M. R., Hood K., Houston, H., Pill, R., Fay, J. and Evans, H. M. (2004) 'Public Attitudes Towards the Use of Primary Care Patient Record Data in Medical Research without Consent: A Qualitative Study', *Journal of Medical Ethics* 30: 104–9.

Rosenthal, R. and Rosnow, R. L. (1969) *Artifact and Behavioural Research*. New York: Academic Press.

Rosnow, R. L. (1990) 'Teaching Research Ethics through Role-Play and Discussion', *Teaching of Psychology* 17(3): 179–81.

Rosnow, R. L., Rotherham-Borus, M.J., Ceci, S. J., Blanck, P. D. and Koocher, G. P. (1993) 'The Institutional Review Board as a Mirror of Scientific and Ethical Standards', *American Psychologist* 48(7): 821–6.

Rothman, D. J. and Rothman, S. M. (1984) *The Willowbrook Wars*. New York: Harper and Row.

Sachs, M. L. (1993) 'Professional Ethics in Sport Psychology', in R. N. Singer, M. Murphey and L. K. Tennant (1993) *Handbook of Research on Sport Psychology*. New York: Macmillan, pp. 921–32.

Sartorius, R. (ed.) (1983) *Paternalism*. Minneapolis, MN: University of Minnesota Press.

Sartre, J.-P. (2003) *Being and Nothingness: An Essay on Phenomenological Ontology*. London: Routledge.

Savulescu, J. (2001) 'Harm, Ethics Committees and the Gene Therapy Death', *Journal of Medical Ethics* 27: 148–50.

Scocozza, L. (1989) 'Ethics and Medical Science: On Voluntary Participation in Biomedical Experimentation', *Acta Sociologica* 32(3): 283–93.

Shaw, S. *et al.* (2005) 'Research Governance: Where Did it Come From? What Does it Mean?', *Journal of the Royal Society of Medicine* 98: 496–502.

Shephard, R. J. (1995) 'Exercise and Sudden Death: An Overview', *Sport Science Review* 4(2): 1–13.

Shephard, R. J. (2002) 'Ethics in Exercise Science Research', *Sports Medicine* 32 (3): 169–83.

Sherman, N. (1989) *The Fabric of Character*. Oxford: Clarendon Press.

Shrader-Frechette, K. (1994) *Ethics of Scientific Research*. Lanham, MD: Rowman and Littlefield.

Sieber, J. E. (1992) *Planning Ethically Responsible Research*. London: Sage.

Sieber, J. E. (1998) 'The Psychology of Whistleblowing', *Science and Engineering Ethics* 4: 7–23.

Singer, P. (ed.) (1993) *A Companion to Ethics*. Oxford: Blackwell.

Skinner, A. (1998) 'In NHS Appointments, Research Output Should not be Used as Yardstick of Ability', *British Medical Journal* 317(1590).

Skorupski, J. (1991) *John Stuart Mill*. London: Routledge.

Smith, R. (1998) 'The Need for a National Body for Research Misconduct', *British Medical Journal* 316: 1686–7.

Smith, R. (2005) Investigating the Previous Studies of a Fraudulent Author', *British Medical Journal* 331: 288–91.

Solomon, R. C. (1993) *Ethics and Excellence*. Oxford: Oxford University Press.

Sparkes, A. C. (1992) 'The Paradigms Debate: An Extended Review and a Celebration of Difference', in A. Sparkes (ed.) *Research in Physical Education and Sport: Exploring Alternative Visions*. London: Falmer Press, pp. 9–60.

Sparkes, A. C. (1996) 'The Fatal Flaw: A Narrative of the Fragile Body Self', *Qualitative Inquiry* 2: 463–94.

Sparkes, A. C. (1998) 'Validity in Qualitative Inquiry and the Problem of Criteria: Implications for Sports Psychology', *The Sports Psychologist* 12: 363–86.

Sparkes, A. C. (2000) 'Autoethnography and Narratives of the Self', *Sociology of Sport Journal* 17(2): 21–43.

Sparkes, A. C. (2002) *Telling Tales in Sport and Physical Activity*. Leeds: Human Kinetics.

Sparkes, A. C. and Smith, B. (2003) 'Men, Sport, Spinal Cord Injury and Narrative Time', *Qualitative Research* 2: 295–320.

Spriggs, M. (2004) 'Canaries in the Mines: Children, Risk, Non-Therapeutic Research and Justice', *Journal of Medical Ethics* 30: 176–81.

Stetten, D. (1975) 'Freedom of Inquiry', *Science* 189(4207): 953.

Stewart, H. (2002) 'Harms, Wrongs, and Set-Backs in Feinberg's Moral Limits of the Criminal Law', *Buffalo Criminal Law Review* 15: 47–67.

Stone, T. H. (2003) 'The Invisible Vulnerable', *Journal of Law, Medicine and Ethics* 31(1): 149–53.

Sugden, J. (1995) 'Fieldworkers Rush In (Where Theorists Fear to Tread): The Perils of Ethnography', in A. Tomlinson, and S. Fleming (eds) *Ethics, Sport and Leisure: Crises and Critiques*. Brighton: CSRC, pp. 223–44.

Sugden, J. (2002) *Scum Airways: Inside Football's Underground Economy*. London: Mainstream.

Sugden, J. (2005) 'Is Investigative Sociology Just Investigative Journalism?', in M. J. McNamee (ed.) *Philosophy and the Sciences of Exercise, Health and Sport*. London: Routledge, pp. 203–18.

Swain, J. B. *et al.* (1998) 'Public Research, Private Concerns: Ethical Issues in the Use of Open-Ended Interviews with People Who Have Learning Difficulties', *Disability and Society* 13(1): 21–36.

Taylor, C. (1985) *Philosophy and the Human Sciences*. Cambridge: Cambridge University Press.

Tickle, L. (2002) 'Opening Windows, Closing Doors: Ethical Dilemmas in Educational Action Research', in M. J. McNamee and D. Bridges (eds) *Ethics and Educational Research*. Oxford: Blackwell, pp. 41–57.

Tolfrey, K., Campbell, I. G. and Jones A. M. (1999) 'Intra-individual Variation of Plasma Lipids and Lipoproteins in Prepubescent Children', *European Journal of Applied Physiology and Occupational Physiology* 79(5): 449–56.

Toulmin, S. E. (2001) *Return to Reason*. Boston, MA: Harvard University Press.

Tronto, J. C. (1993) *Moral Boundaries: A Political Argument for an Ethic of Care*. London: Routledge.

Truss, L. (2003) *Eats, Shoots and Leaves: The Zero Tolerance Approach to Punctuation*. London: Profile

Tsalis, G., Nikolaidis, M. G. and Mougios, V. (2004) 'Effects of Iron Intake through Food or Supplement on Iron Status and Performance of Healthy Adolescent Swimmers during a Training Season', *International Journal of Sports Medicine* 25(4): 306–13.

Tully, J., Ninis, N., Booy, R. and Viner, R. (2000) 'The New System of Multicentre Research Ethics Committees: Prospective Study', *British Medical Journal* 320(7243): 1179–81.

USA Federal and Institutional Guidelines (2005) URL: http://www.hhs.gov/ohrp/humansubjects/guidance/45cfr46.htm, accessed 7 March 2006.

Veatch, R. M. (ed.) (1989) *Medical Ethics*. Boston, MA: Jones and Bartlett Publishers.

Verity, C. and Nicholl, A. (2002) 'Consent, Confidentially and the Threat to Public Health Surveillance', *British Medical Journal* 324: 1210–13.

Waldron, J. (ed.) (1989) *Theories of Rights*. Oxford: Oxford University Press.

Wallace, P., Haines, A., Harrison, R., Barber, J., Thompson, S., Jacklin, P. *et al.* (2002a) 'Joint Teleconsultations (Virtual Outreach) Versus Standard Outpatient Appointments for Patients Referred by their General Practitioner for a Specialist Opinion: A Randomised Trial', *The Lancet* 359(9322): 1961–8.

Wallace, P., Haines, A., Harrison, R., Barber, J. A., Thompson, S., Roberts, J. *et al.* (2002b) 'Design and Performance of a Multi-centre Randomised Controlled Trial and Economic Evaluation of Joint Teleconsultations', *BMC Family Practice* 3: 1.

Waller, J. (2002) *Fabulous Science*. Oxford: Oxford University Press.

Walley, T. (2006) 'Using Personal Health Information in Medical Research', *British Medical Journal* 332: 130–1.

WAME (World Association of Medical Editors) (2005) 'Ghost Writing Initiated by Commercial Companies'. URL: http://www.wame.org/wamestmt.htm#ghost, accessed 16 Jan. 2006.

Watson, J. D. and Crick, F. H. C. (1953) 'Genetic implications of the structure of deoxyribonucleic acid', *Nature* 171 (4361): 964–7.

Weinberg, M.S. (1968) 'Embarrassment: Its Variable and Invariable Aspects', *Social Forces* 46(3): 382–8.

Wellcome Trust (2004) 'DNA Fingerprinting and National DNA Databases'. URL: http://www.wellcome.ac.uk/en/genome/genesandbody/hg07f007.html, accessed 28 Jan. 2006.

White, B. (1992) *Competence to Consent*. Washington, DC: Georgetown University Press.

White, C. (2004) 'Three Journals Raise Doubts on Validity of Canadian Studies', *British Medical Journal* 328: 67.

Whyte, W. F. (1943). *Street Corner Society: The Social Structure of an Italian Slum*. Chicago, IL: University of Chicago Press.

Williams, B. A. O. (1972) *Ethics*. New York: Harper Torchbooks.

Williams, B. A. O. (1985) *Ethics and the Limits of Philosophy*. London: Fontana.

Wittgenstein, L. (1953) *Philosophical Investigations*. Oxford: Blackwell.

WMA (World Medical Association) (2000) *Ethical Principles for Medical Research Involving Human Subjects* (Declaration of Helsinki). France: WMA.

WMA (World Medical Association) (2002) 'WMA International Code of Medical Ethics'. URL: http://www.wma.net/e/policy/c8.htm, accessed July 2006.

Woolf, P. K. (1985) 'Pressure to Publish and Fraud in Science', *Annals of Internal Medicine* 104: 99–102.

Woo-suk, H. (2004) 'Evidence of a Pluripotent Human Embryonic Stem Cell Line Derived from a Cloned Blastocyst', *Science* 303(5664): 1669–74.

Wynands, J. E. (1998) 'Harold Randall Griffith, MD, CM, OC – 1894–1985', Canadian Anesthesiologists' Society. URL: http://www.cas.ca/public/anesthesia_greats/default.asp?load=griffith, accessed 29 Jan. 2006.

Yeadon, M. R. and Morlock, M. (1989) 'The Appropriate Use of Regression Equations for the Estimation of Segmental Inertia Parameters', *Journal of Biomechanics* 22: 683–9.

Zawadzki, Z. and Abbasi, A. (1998) 'Polish Plagiarism Scandal Unearthed', *British Medical Journal* 316: 645.

Zelaznik, H. (1993) 'Ethical Issues in Conducting and Reporting Research: A Response to Matt, Safrit, and Kroll', *Quest* 45(1): 62–8.

Zeller, R. A. (1993) 'Focus Group Research on Sensitive Topics: Setting the Agenda without Setting the Agenda', in D. L. Morgan (ed.) *Successful Focus Groups: Advancing the State of the Art*. London: Sage.

Index

British Association for Sport and Exercise Sciences (BASES) 27, 58, 62, 76, 77, 87, 134
British Medical Association (BMA) 19, 149, 155, 163, 197n2
British Paediatric Association (BPA) 157, 163; *see also* Royal College of Paediatric and Child Health
British Psychological Society (BPS) 134
British Sociological Association (BSA) 27, 134, 196n4
British Sociological Association 58
Brodie, D.A. 12, 54, 72

Capron, A.M. 10, 15, 18, 19, 20, 21, 28
captive populations 23; *see also* voluntariness
Cardinal, B.J. 85
Cardon, P.V. 15
Carrington, B. 161
Casarett, D.J. 53
Cashmore, E. 161
casuistry 46–8, 65
Charlton, J.I. 161, 171
children: protecting 155–6; research on 154–5; therapeutic and non-therapeutic research 159–60; and venepuncture 156–9
Childress, J.F. 42–3, 73–4, 76, 80, 84, 198n2, 198m8
Christakis, N.A. 8, 169, 174, 180
Clarke, G. 140, 146
Code of Federal Regulations 14, 16, 49
codes of conduct 2, 3, 7, 58, 134, 147; regulation by 61–3; vulnerable populations 153–4
Committee for International Organizations of Medical Sciences (CIOMS) 2–3, 5, 51, 52, 149, 155, 158, 160–1, 163, 166, 182–3, 184, 189
Committee on Publication Ethics 126
confidentiality 3, 17, 61, 91, 97–100, 136, 183; associated benefits and harms 103–6; and qualitative research 141–5
consequentialism 33, 34–7, 123, 127, 183
Crandell, R. 26, 84
Crigger, N.J. 167, 169, 174, 175
Crosby, S. 170
Crossett, T. 139
Culver, C.M. 75
Cunliffe, J. 130

D'Agostino, F. 26
data: collection 3, 4, 54, 184, 189; storage 98, 136; *see also* anonymity
Data Protection Act 81, 92, 102

Davis, M. 122–3
Dawson, A.J. 26
Dawson, N. 166, 167, 170, 175, 180
deceptive research 4, 61, 133, 135, 139–40
Declaration of Helsinki 2, 25, 51, 52, 53, 72, 149, 155, 157, 158, 163
deontology 32–3, 152; *see also* duty-based moral theories
Department of Health 50, 51; Research Governance Framework 50
Department of Health and Human Services (DHHS) 27, 54
Department of Health, Employment and Welfare (DHEW) 14, 27
Dickert, N. 82, 83
Diener, E. 26, 84
Disability Rights Movement (DRM) 161
Drowatzky, J.N. 4
duty-based moral theory 2, 11, 33, 37–8; codes of conduct 61
Dworkin, G. 70
Dyer, C. 120
Dyer, O. 121

Eaton, L. 116
Economic and Social Research Council (ESRC) 9, 134
Edwards, S.D. 81, 159, 200n1, 200n3, 201n1
Edwards, S.J.L. 190, 191
Elias, N. 95
Embassy of France in the US 92
English Institute of Sport 28
Environmental Protection Agency 124
Eraut, M. 125, 199n11
European Clinical Trials Directive 28, 50
European College of Sports Science (ECSS) 58
Evans, D. 12, 156, 159
Evans, M. 12, 156, 159

Faden, R.R. 19, 20, 22, 23, 24, 26, 175, 176
Fairchild, A. 163
Feinburg, J. 70, 103
feminist ethics 39–40
Fethe, C. 12
Fine, G. 139
Fishwick, L. 135, 143
Flynn, S. 64
Food and Drug Administration (FDA) 15, 27
Foucault, M. 93
French, E. 12, 166, 171, 176
Friedson, E. 201n8

Royal College of Paediatric and Child
    Health (RCPCH) 5, 149, 155, 157, 158,
    163
Royal College of Physicians 27

Sachs, M.L. 141
Sartorius, R. 70
Sartre, J.P. 96
Savulescu, J. 190, 191
scientific method 4, 110, 196n1
scientific misconduct 109–11
Scocozza, L. 11, 12
Shaw, S. 49
Shephard, R.J. 84, 146, 154, 194
Sherman, N. 199n7
Sieber, J.E. 73, 125, 199n9
Singer, P. 34, 197n2
Skinner, A. 127, 128
Skorupski, J. 68
Smith, B. 138
Smith, R. 125
Solomon, R.C. 37
Sparkes, A.C. 8, 132, 138, 143, 145,
    146
Sport and Exercise Science of New
    Zealand (SESNZ) Association 75
Spriggs, M. 149, 159
Stetten, D. 64
Stewart, D. 44
Stewart, H. 103
Stone, T.H. 161
Stopani, K. 12, 54, 72
straightforward application model *see*
    Rachels, J.
subjectivism 2, 40–1
Sugden, J. 41, 75, 135, 136, 141
Swain, J.B. 140, 147
Szasz, T. 153

Taylor, C. 201n6
teleology 32–3
Thacker, P.G. 82
therapeutic and non-therapeutic research
    10, 15, 25, 196n3, 197n8; and children
    159–60; *see also* children
Tickle, L. 141, 201n5
Tolfrey, K. 158
Toulmin, S.E. 4, 46, 110
Tronto, J.C. 39
Troyna, B. 161
trust 4; *see also* vulnerable populations
Tsalis, G. 158

Tulley, J. 64
Tuskegee experiments 13, 163

universality 173–6
utilitarianism 11, 12, 34–7, 142, 200–1n6;
    act and rule utilitarianism 36; *see also*
    consequentialism

validity 8, 132
Vancouver Guidelines 114
Veatch, R.M. 44, 71, 88
venepuncture 5, 200n6; *see also* children
Verity, C. 102
virtue-based moral theory 11, 33, 39–40,
    109, 164; moral virtues and practices
    128–9
voluntariness 73; and captive populations
    78–80; and gatekeepers 80; and
    payment 82–4; *see also* informed
    consent
vulnerable populations 4, 17, 89, 138;
    power and trust 140–1, 149–53; *see also*
    codes of conduct, children

Waldron, J. 38
Wallace, P. 120
Waller, J. 198n2
Walley, T. 102
Weinburg, M.S. 96
Wellcome Trust 101
whistleblowing 4, 122–6, 199n10, 199n11
White, B. 198n6
White, C. 125
Whtye, W.F. 138
Williams, B.A.O. 32, 36, 46
Wittgenstein, L. 62
Woolf, P.K. 198n1
Woo-suk, H. 121–2
World Association of Medical Editors
    (WAME) 115–16
World Health Organization (WHO) 4–5;
    Research Ethics Review Committee 153
World Medical Association (WMA) 2,
    25, 196n3
Wynands, J.E. 190

Yeadon, M.R. 154

Zawadski, Z. 119
Zelaznik, H. 17, 18, 23, 65, 140, 143
Zeller, R.A. 102
Zimbardo, P. 24